Manual for Eye Examination and Diagnosis

Mark W. Leitman, MD

Clinical Assistant Professor
Department of Ophthalmology and Visual Sciences
Montefiore Hospital
Albert Einstein College of Medicine
Bronx, NY, USA

Attending Physician
St. Peter's Medical Center
New Brunswick, NJ, USA

NINTH EDITION

WILEY Blackwell

Published by John Wiley & Sons, Inc., Hoboken, New Jersey
Published simultaneously in Canada

For general information on our other products and services or for technical support, please contact our Customer Care Department within the United States at (800) 762-2974, outside the United States at (317) 572-3993 or fax (317) 572-4002.

Wiley also publishes its books in a variety of electronic formats. Some content that appears in print may not be available in electronic formats. For more information about Wiley products, visit our web site at www.wiley.com.

Library of Congress Cataloging-in-Publication Data:

Names: Leitman, Mark W., 1946-, author.
Title: Manual for eye examination and diagnosis / Mark W. Leitman.
Description: Ninth edition. | Hoboken, New Jersey : John Wiley & Sons Inc.,
   [2016] | Includes bibliographical references and index.
Identifiers: LCCN 2016003738 | ISBN 9781119243618 (pbk.) | ISBN 9781119243632
   (Adobe PDF) | ISBN 9781119243625 (ePub)
Subjects: | MESH: Eye Diseases--diagnosis | Diagnostic Techniques,
   Ophthalmological | Handbooks
Classification: LCC RE75 | NLM WW 39 | DDC 617.7/15--dc23 LC record available at http://lccn.loc.gov/2016003738

Cover image: Julia Monsenego, CRA, Wills Eye Hospital and Carl Zeiss Meditec, Inc.

10 9 8 7 6 5 4 3 2 1

A serious student is like a seed:
with so much potential it will grow
almost anywhere it lands.

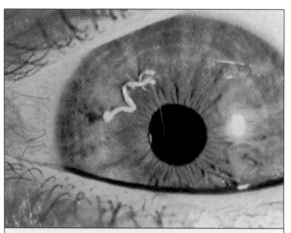

Fig. I A seed introduced into the eye of an 8 year-old boy through a penetrating corneal wound became imbedded in the iris. Many months later, the seed became visible when it began germinating. Courtesy of Solomon Abel, MD, FRCS, DOMS, and *Arch. Ophthalmol.*, Sept. 1979, Vol. 97, p. 1651.

Contents

Preface

The first edition of this book was started when I was a medical student 44 years ago during the allotted 2-week rotation in the eye clinic. It was published during my first year of eye residency with assistance and encouragement from my chairman, Dr Paul Henkind. At that time, all introductory books were 500 pages or more and could not be read quickly enough to understand what was going on. With this in mind, each word of this 175-page practical manual was carefully chosen so that students understand the refraction and hundreds of the most commonly encountered eye diseases from the onset. They are discussed with respect to anatomy, instrumentation, differential diagnosis, and treatment in the order in which they would be uncovered during the eye exam and are highlighted with 551 photos and illustrations.

The book is meant to be read in its entirety in several hours and, hopefully, impart to you a foundation on which to grow and enjoy this beautiful and ever-changing specialty. The popularity of previous editions has resulted in translations into Spanish, Japanese, Indonesian, Italian, Russian, Greek, Polish, and Portuguese, and an Indian reprint.

My special appreciation goes to Johnson & Johnson eye care division, which provided a generous grant to distribute the seventh edition to 40,000 students. I sponsored the eighth edition, and this newest ninth edition, with distribution to 69,000 medical students. Many images were generously provided by Pfizer's website, Xalatan.com, several journals, Wills Eye Hospital, the University of Iowa, Montefiore Hospital, and many colleagues. Elliot Davidoff, who sat next to me in medical school, and who is now Assistant Professor at the Ohio State University, surprised me with many unsolicited contributions, as did medical student, Lance Lyons.

This edition has been updated with 50 new images. I hope you enjoy reading it half as much as I enjoyed writing it. I have received no monetary funding from and I have no association with any company whose products are mentioned in this book.

I would appreciate any recommendations and images that would improve the next edition. You may email me at mark.leitman@aol.com.

MARK W. LEITMAN

Introduction to the eye team and their instruments

The eye exam depends on many sophisticated, and costly instruments, together with highly trained professionals to operate them.

Ophthalmologist The ophthalmologist attended 4 years of college, 4 years of medical (MD) or osteopathic (DO) school, and 3 years of specialty eye residency training. They may remain general ophthalmologists, but now, more often than not, spend an additional 1–2 years subspecializing in corneal and external disease, vitreoretinal disease, cataracts, glaucoma, neuro-ophthalmology, oculoplastic surgery, pathology, pediatric (strabismus), or uveitis. They often employ three allied health professionals. Ophthalmologists perform all aspects of eye care. They are the sole professional allowed to perform laser and other ocular surgeries. There are five lasers of different wavelengths. Argon lasers are used to treat glaucoma and retinal disease, most commonly diabetic retinopathy. Nd:YAG lasers are usually used to open secondary cataracts after cataract extractions and to perform peripheral iridotomies for narrow-angle glaucoma. Excimer lasers reshape the cornea in the refraction procedure called LASIK. Femtosecond lasers may replace certain manual parts of routine cataract extractions. Carbon dioxide lasers are utilized for dermatologic procedures.

Optometrist (OD) The optometrist completes 4 years of college and 4 years of optometry school. They perform similar tasks to the ophthalmologist, with the exception of surgery. They may establish their own practice or work for an ophthalmologist. Subspecialities often include pediatrics and low vision.

Opticians (ABO, American Board of Opticians) Opticians grind the lenses and put them in frames (laboratory optician) or fit them on the patient (dispensing optician). Their training and certification is highly variable from state to state, but often includes 2 years at a community college.

Ocularists (BCO, BRDO, FASO) There are no schools to teach this craft. These technicians learn by apprenticeship. They then have to pass tests for certification. They fit the scleral shell needed after removal of an eye (Fig. 395).

Ophthalmic technicians Ophthalmic technicians have varying degrees of licensure. With medical supervision, they may take medical histories; measure eye pressure; do refractions and visual field testing; take visual activities; teach contact lens fitting; and perform fluorescein angiography to study retinal blood flow. Technicians use an optical coherence tomography (OCT) instrument to measure each layer of the eye and the blood vessels by reflecting light off the intraocular structures. This requires a clear medium, as opposed to ultrasound which utilizes reflective sound waves. To appreciate the precision of ophthalmic testing and procedures one must realize a red blood cell is 7 µm (micrometers) in diameter. OCT measures 5 µm changes in the retinal thickness to evaluate edema and glaucoma loss using 30,000 A-scans per second. A surgically created LASIK flap is 110 µm (Figs 59 and 60) and an epi-LASIK flap (Fig. 67) is only 30 µm. A-scan ultrasound measures the length of the eye needed to determine the power of an intraocular lens used in cataract surgery and B-scan ultrasound measures individual layers. Ultrasound is useful with opaque media that limit direct visualization or OCT testing.

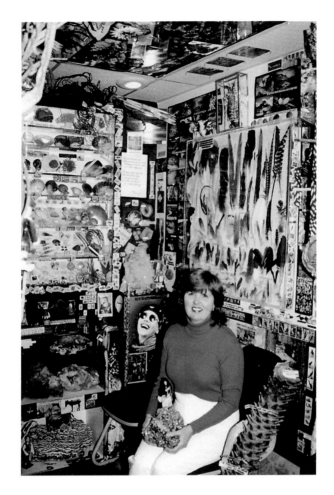

Dedicated to Andrea Kase

It is impossible to perform a good eye exam without a good support team. Andrea has enthusiastically led our team for 35 years as office manager, ophthalmic technician, and typist of all correspondence, including the last seven editions of this book. By encouraging me to bring my collection of rocks and other objects from nature into the waiting room, she helped create a museum that my patients look forward to seeing.

Chapter 1
Medical history

The history includes the patient's chief complaints, medical illnesses, current medications, allergies to medications, and family history of eye disease.

Common chief complaints	Causes
Persistent loss of vision	**1** Focusing problems are the most common complaints. Everyone eventually needs glasses to attain perfect vision, and fitting lenses occupies half the eye care professional's day.
	2 Cataracts are cloudy lenses that occur in everyone in later life. Unoperated cataracts are the leading cause of blindness worldwide. In the USA, over 3.3 million cataract extractions are performed each year.
	3 Thirteen percent of American adults are treated for diabetes. Another 40% are pre-diabetic. It is the leading cause of blindness in the USA in those under 65 years of age.
	4 Age-related macular degeneration (AMD) causes loss of central vision and is the leading cause of blindness in people over age 65. Signs are present in 25% of people over age 75, increasing to almost 100% by age 100.
	5 Glaucoma is a disease of the optic nerve that is usually due to elevated eye pressure. It mostly occurs after age 35 and affects 2 million Americans, with black persons affected five times as often as white persons. Peripheral vision is lost first, with no symptoms until it is far advanced. This is why routine eye exams are recommended.
Transient loss of vision lasting less than ½ hour, with or without flashing lights	In younger patients, think of migrainous spasm of cerebral arteries. With aging, consider emboli from arteriosclerotic plaques.
Floaters	Almost everyone will at some time see shifting spots due to suspended particles in the normally clear vitreous. They are usually physiologic, but may result from hemorrhage, retinal detachments, or other serious conditions.
Flashes of light (photopsia)	The retina accounts for 84% of complaints, which are usually unilateral. Simple sparks are most often due to vitreous traction on the retina (Fig. 523). Insults to the visual center in the brain (16%) are most often migrainous, but ministrokes, especially in the elderly, must be considered. Cerebral causes are often bilateral, with more formed images, such as zigzag lines (Fig. 133).

Continued on p. 2

Manual for Eye Examination and Diagnosis, Ninth edition. Mark Leitman.
© 2017 John Wiley & Sons, Inc. Published 2017 by John Wiley & Sons, Inc.

Common chief complaints	Causes
Night blindness (nyctalopia)	Nyctalopia usually indicates a need for spectacle change, but also commonly occurs with aging and cataracts. Rarer causes include retinitis pigmentosa and vitamin A deficiency.
Double vision (diplopia)	Strabismus, which affects 4% of the population, is the condition where the eyes do not look in the same direction. This binocular diplopia disappears when one eye is covered. In straight-eyed persons, diplopia is often confused with blurry vision or caused by hysteria or a beam-splitting opacity in one eye that does not disappear by covering the other eye.
Light sensitivity (photophobia)	Usually, a normal condition treated with tinted lenses, but could result from inflammation of the eye or brain; internal reflection of light in lightly pigmented or albinotic eyes; or dispersion of light by mucous, lens, and corneal opacities, or retinal degeneration.
Itching	Most often due to allergy and dry eye.
Headache	Headache patients present daily to rule out eye causes and to seek direction.
	1 Headache due to blurred vision or eye-muscle imbalance worsens with the use of eyes.
	2 Tension causes 80–90% of headaches. They typically worsen with anxiety and are often associated with bilateral temple and neck pain.
	3 Migraine occurs in 18% of women and 6% of men. This recurrent pounding headache, often lasting for hours, but less than a day, is sometimes accompanied by nausea, bilateral blurred vision, and flashing, zigzag lights. It is relieved by sleep and may be aggravated by bright light and certain foods.
	4 Sinusitis causes a dull ache about the eyes and occasional tenderness over a sinus (Fig. 207). There may be an associated nasal stuffiness and a history of allergy.
	5 Menstrual headaches are cyclical.
	6 Sharp ocular pains lasting for seconds are often referred from nerve irritations in the neck, nasal mucosa, or intracranial dura, which, like the eye, are also innervated by the trigeminal nerve.
	7 Headaches that awaken the patient and are prolonged or associated with focal neurologic symptoms should be referred for neurologic study.
Visual hallucinations	These most often occur in the elderly, especially in those with dementia, psychosis, or reduced sensory stimulation, as in blindness and deafness. Many medications, including cephalosporins, sulfa drugs, dopamines used to treat Parkinson's disease, vasoconstrictors, or vasodilators should be considered.
Increased tearing (epiphora)	Consider increased production due to emotion and eye irritation or decreased ability of a normally generated tear to drain into the nose.

Medical illnesses

Record all systemic diseases. Diabetes and thyroid disease are two that are most commonly associated with eye disease.

Diabetes mellitus

1 Diabetes (see Front cover image) may be first diagnosed when there are large changes in spectacle correction causing blurriness. It is due to the effect of blood sugar changes on the lens of the eye.

2 Diabetes is one of the common causes of III, IV, and VI cranial nerve paralysis. It is due to closure of brainstem vessels. The resulting diplopia may be the first symptom of diabetes and often resolves by 10 weeks.

3 Retinopathy due to microvascular disease may result in macular edema. It is the primary reason for blindness before age 65. Patients with diabetes should have annual eye exams, because early treatment is critical. As retinopathy is rare in children, most Type 1 diabetic screenings may be delayed until a child is 15, or 5 years after diagnosis.

Autoimmune (Graves') thyroid disease

This is a condition in which an orbitopathy may be present with hyper- but also hypo- or euthyroid disease.

1 It is the most common cause of bulging eyes, referred to as exophthalmos (proptosis). This is due to fibroblast proliferation and mucopolysaccharide infiltration of the orbit. A small white area of sclera appearing between the lid and upper cornea is diagnostic of thyroid disease 90% of the time (Figs 1 and 2). This exposed sclera may be a result of exophthalmos or thyroid lid retraction due to stimulation of Müller's muscle that elevates the lid. Severe orbitopathy may be treated with steroids, radiation, or surgical decompression of the orbit (Fig. 3).

2 Infiltration of eye muscles may cause diplopia, which is confirmed by a computed tomography (CT) scan (Figs 2 and 3).

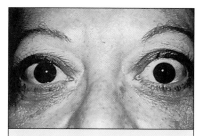

Fig. 1 Thyroid exophthalmos with exposed sclera at superior limbus.

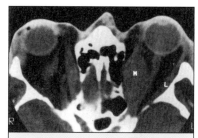

Fig. 2 CT scan of thyroid orbitopathy showing filtration of medial rectus muscle (M) and normal lateral rectus muscle (L). Compression of left optic nerve could cause optic neuropathy. This is called crowded apex syndrome. Courtesy of Jack Rootman.

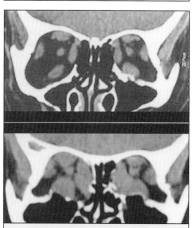

Fig. 3 Orbital CT scan of Graves' orbitopathy before surgical decompression (above) and after right orbital floor osteotomy (below). Often three, but rarely all four, bony walls may be opened. Note thickened extraocular muscles. Courtesy of Lelio Baldeschi, MD, and *Ophthalmology*, July 2007, Vol. 114, pp. 1395–1402.

3 Exophthalmos may cause excessive exposure of the eye in the day and an inability to close the lids at night (lagophthalmos), resulting in corneal dessication.

4 Optic nerve compression is the worst complication and occurs in 4% of patients with thyroid disease. It could cause permanent loss of vision (Fig. 2) and immediate intravenous steroids should be considered when vision is threatened.

Medications (ocular side effects)

Record patient medications. Those taking the following commonly prescribed drugs are often referred to an eye doctor to monitor ocular side effects.

Hydroxychloroquine (Plaquenil), initially used to treat malaria, is now a cornerstone medication used to treat autoimmune diseases, such as rheumatoid arthritis, lupus erythematosus, and Sjögren's syndrome. It may cause "bull's eye" maculopathy (Fig. 4) and corneal deposits. Patients should get a baseline eye exam before starting medication. It includes visual acuity, Amsler grid, color vision, and examination of the retina to rule out pre-exisiting maculopathy. The patient should follow-up every 6 months. Depending on the dosage and the chronicity of use, the eye doctor will determine if additional tests are necessary. Risk increases if dosage exceeds 6.5 mg/kg, especially when taken for more than 5 years and if there is pre-existing macular degeneration. These high-dose patients may also have routine monitoring of their peripheral visual fields and optical coherence tomography (OCT) testing for parafoveal retinal pigment epithelial cell damage.

The retina is also adversely affected by phenothiazine tranquilizers (Fig. 5); niacin, a lipid-lowering agent; tamoxifen, used for breast cancer (Figs 6–8); and interferon used to treat multiple sclerosis and hepatitis C.

Ethambutol, rifampin, isoniazid, streptomycin – taken mainly for tuberculosis – may all cause optic neuropathy. The antidepressants

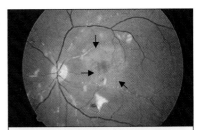

Fig. 4 Bull's eye maculopathy due to hydroxychloroquine in a patient with systemic lupus. The vasculitis and white cotton-wool spots are due to the lupus. Courtesy of Russel Rand, MD, and *Arch. Ophthalmol.*, Apr. 2000, Vol. 118, pp. 588–589. Copyright 2000, American Medical Association. All rights reserved.

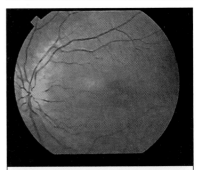

Fig. 5 Phenothiazine maculopathy with pigment mottling of the macula.

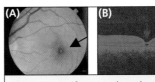

Fig. 6 Tamoxifen maculopathy with crystalline depositis (A); and (B) OCT showing crystals in the fovea. Courtesy of Joao Liporaci, MD.

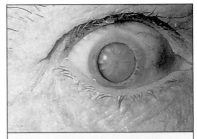

Fig. 7 Tamoxifen causes cataracts.

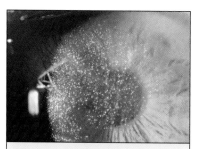

Fig. 8 Besides causing maculopathy and cataracts, tamoxifen also causes crystal deposition in the cornea (keratopathy). Courtesy of Olga Zinchuk, MD, and *Arch. Ophthalmol.*, July 2006, Vol. 124, p. 1046. Copyright 2006, American Medical Association. All rights reserved.

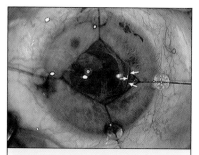

Fig. 9 Iris retractors are one method used to open poorly dilated pupils during cataract surgery. Note edge of lens implant (↑) behind iris. Courtesy of Bonnie Henderson, MD, Harvard Medical School.

Paxil, Prozac, and Zoloft may also cause optic neuropathy. Corticosteroids may cause posterior subcapsular cataracts (Fig. 400), glaucoma, and a reduction in immunity that may increase the incidence of herpes keratitis.

Flomax (tamsulosin), the most common treatment for an enlarged prostate gland, increases the complications in cataract surgery by decreasing the ability to dilate the pupil, a condition referred to as intraoperative floppy iris syndrome (IFIS). Pupillary expansion devices (Fig. 9) and additional pupillary dilating medications usually prevent complications.

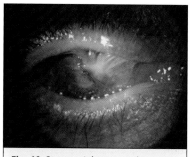

Fig. 10 Stevens–Johnson syndrome with inflammation and adhesions of lid and bulbar conjunctiva. Reprinted with permission from *Am. J. Ophthalmol.*, Aug. 2008, Vol. 1146, p. 271. Surgical strategies for fornix reconstruction. Based on *Symblepharon Severity*, Ahmad Kheirhah, Gabriella Blanco, Victoria Casas, Yasutaka Hayashida, Vadrecu K. Radu, Scheffer C.G. Tseng. Copyright 2008, Elsevier.

Stevens–Johnson syndrome (Fig. 10) is an immunologic reaction to a foreign substance, usually drugs, and most commonly sulfonamides, barbiturates, and penicillin. Some 100 other medications have also been implicated. It often affects the skin and mucous membranes. It could be fatal in 35% of cases.

Prostaglandin analogues are the most commonly prescribed glaucoma medications. They may irreversibly darken the iris (Fig. 11) with reversible lengthening and darkening of the eyelashes and skin of the lids (Fig. 13). The side effect of longer, darker lashes has gener-

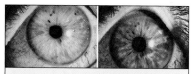

Fig. 11 Irreversible darkening of a blue iris after 3 months of latanoprost (Xalatan) therapy. This is the most common drug for treating glaucoma. Courtesy of N. Pfeiffer, MD, P. Appleton, MD, and *Arch. Ophthalmol.*, Feb 2011, Vol. 119, p. 191. Copyright 2001, American Medical Association. All rights reserved.

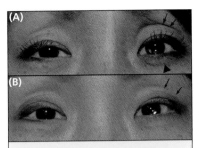

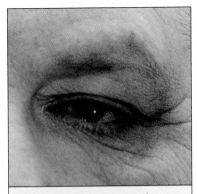

Fig. 12 (A) Prostaglandin-analogue-induced fat atrophy of the left orbit with sunken superior sulcus after 1 year (↑) and darkened skin (^). Courtesy of University of Iowa, Eyerounds.org. (B) After discontinuing eye drops that had been used in the left eye for 1 year, orbital fat atrophy, darkened and lengthened lashes, and improved skin pigmentation are seen. Courtesy of N. Pfeiffer, MD, P. Appleton, MD, and *Arch. Ophthalmol.*, Feb 2011, Vol. 119, p. 191. Copyright 2001, American Medical Association. All rights reserved.

Fig. 13 After long-term use of prostaglandin analogue in the left eye, the patient developed hyperpigmentation of periorbital skin, darkening and lengthening of lashes, and loss of orbital fat, causing a deepening of the upper eyelid sulcus.

ated a drug: Latisse. It is applied once a day to the upper eyelid lashes for cosmetic reasons. This group of drugs may also reduce orbital fat, causing a sunken upper lid sulcus (Fig. 12).

Amiodarone (Cordarone, Pacerone), one of the most potent anti-arrhythmia drugs, and sildenafil (Viagra), tadalafil (Cialis), and vardenafil (Levitra), used to treat erectile dysfunction, have all been suspected of causing nonarteritic anterior ischemic optic neuropathy. Amiodarone almost always causes deposits in the cornea that rarely reduce vision, but may cause glare (Fig. 14).

Allergies to medications

Inquire about drug allergies before eye drops are placed or medications prescribed. Neomycin, a popular antibiotic eye drop, may cause conjunctivitis and reddened skin (Fig. 15).

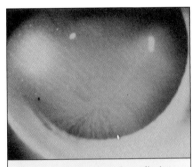

Fig. 14 Epithelial deposits radiating from a central point in the inferior cornea. They occur in almost all patients with Fabry's disease, which is an X-linked systemic accumulation of a glycosphingolipid. Easily seen on a slit lamp exam, it can be the first clue in recognizing the presence of this disease, which is amenable to therapy. Indistinguishable deposits eventually appear in almost all patients using amiodarone and with hydroxychloroquine. Courtesy of Neal A. Sher, MD, and *Arch. Ophthalmol.*, Aug. 1979, Vol. 97, pp. 671–676. Copyright 1979. American Medical Association. All rights reserved.

Family history of eye disease

Cataracts, refractive errors, retinal degeneration, and strabismus – to name a few – may all be inherited. In glaucoma, family members have a 10% chance of acquiring the disease. Eighty percent of people with migraine have an immediate relative with the disease.

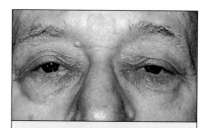

Fig. 15 Neomycin allergy occurs in 5–10% of the population.

> A special question should be directed to the smoking of cigarettes since it doubles the rate of cataracts, macular degeneration, and all types of uveitis. It also worsens exophthalmos in thyroid disease. Cigarette smoking and smokeless tobacco use among American adults is about 20%. At age 70, 80% of Americans have high blood pressure. Over 50% of adults are diabetics or pre-diabetic. It is predicted that 1 in 3 children born after the year 2000 will develop Type 2 diabetes. One third of Americans are obese and one third are overweight. Remind patients that a major change in lifestyle is needed to stem the pandemic of these chronic diseases. Patients should be reminded about minimizing consumption of red and preserved meats, salt, sugar, and saturated fats. Recommend instead a diet rich in fruits, vegetables, beans, nuts, fish, and whole-grain cereals. Staying thin, stress reduction, and a routine daily exercise program should also be advocated.

Chapter 2
Measurement of vision and refraction

Visual acuity

A patient should read the Snellen chart (Fig. 16) from 20 ft (6 m) with the left eye occluded first. Take the vision in each eye without and then with spectacles.

Vision is expressed in a fraction-like form. The top number (numerator; usually 20) is the distance in feet at which the patient reads the chart. The bottom number (denominator) is the size of the object seen at that distance. Whenever acuity is less than 20/20, determine the cause for the decreased vision. The most common cause is a refractive error; i.e., the need for lens correction.

If visual acuity is less than 20/20, the patient may be examined with a pinhole. Improvement of vision while looking through a pinhole indicates that spectacles will improve vision.

Use an "E" chart with a young child or an illiterate adult. Ask the patient which way the ∃ is pointing. Near vision is checked with a reading card held at 14 inches (36 cm). If a refraction for new spectacles is necessary, perform it prior to other tests that may disturb the eye.

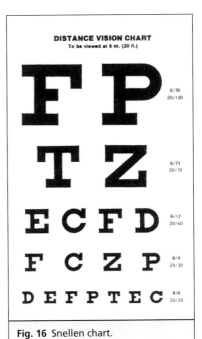

Fig. 16 Snellen chart.

Examples of visual acuity	
Measurement in feet (meters in parentheses)	*Meaning*
20/20 (6/6)	Normal. At 20 ft (6 m), patient reads a line that a normal eye sees at 20 ft.
20/30–2 (6/9–2)	Missed two letters of 20/30 line.
20/50 (6/15)	Vision required in at least one eye for driver's license in most states.

Continued on p. 9

Manual for Eye Examination and Diagnosis, Ninth edition. Mark Leitman.

Continued

Measurement in feet (meters in parentheses)	Meaning
20/200 (6/60)	Legally blind. At 20 ft, patient reads line that normal eye could see at 200 ft (60 m).
10/400 (3/120)	If patient cannot read top line at 20 ft, walk him or her to the chart. Record as the numerator the distance at which the top line first becomes clear.
CF/2ft. (counts fingers at 2 ft, 0.6 m)	If patient is unable to read top line, have the patient count fingers at maximal distance.
HM/3ft (hand motion at 3 ft, 0.9 m)	If at 1 ft (0.3 m) patient cannot count fingers, ask if they see the direction of hand motion.
LP/Proj. (light perception with projection)	Light perception with ability to determine position of the light.
NLP	No light perception: totally blind

Record vision as follows			Key	
$V\!\!\!\!\diagup\!\!\!\!\overline{s}$	OD	20/70 + 1	V	Vision
	OS	LP/Proj.	$\overline{s}$	Without spectacles
			$\overline{c}$	With spectacles
			OD	Right eye
$V\!\!\!\!\diagup\!\!\!\!\overline{c}$	OD	20/20	OS	Left eye
	OS	LP/Proj.	OU	Both eyes

Optics

Emmetropia (no refractive error)

In an emmetropic eye (Fig. 17), light from a distance is focused on the retina.

Ametropia

In this disorder, light is not focused on the retina. The four types are hyperopia, myopia, astigmatism, and presbyopia.

Hyperopia

Parallel rays of light are focused behind the retina (Fig. 18). The patient is farsighted and sees more clearly at a distance than near, but still might require glasses for distance.

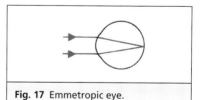

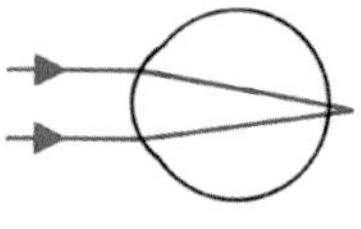

Fig. 17 Emmetropic eye.

Fig. 18 Hyperopic eye.

A convex lens is used to correct hyperopia (Fig. 19). The power of the lens needed to focus incoming light onto the retina is expressed in positive diopters (D). A positive 1 D lens converges parallel rays of light to focus at 1 m (Fig. 20).

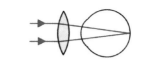

Fig. 19 Hyperopic eye corrected with convex lens.

Myopia

Parallel rays are focused in front of the retina (Fig. 21). The patient is nearsighted and sees more clearly near than at distance. Myopia often begins in the first decade and progresses until stabilization at the end of the second or third decade. A 2016 study – the largest ever done in America – showed that in the past 50 years the prevalence of myopia in young Americans has more than doubled. It has been reported to be as high as 90% in Asia, where, 60 years ago, there was an incidence of 10–20%. It is strongly linked to inheritance, higher levels of education, more near work, less outdoor activity, and not enough sunlight. A concave negative lens (Fig. 22), which diverges light rays, is used to correct this condition.

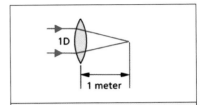

Fig. 20 Parallel rays focused by 1 D lens.

Refractive myopia is due to increased curvature of the cornea or the human lens, whereas axial myopia is due to elongation of the eye. In axial myopia, the retina is sometimes stretched so much that it pulls away from the optic disk (see Fig. 434) and may cause retinal thinning (see Fig. 435) with subsequent holes or detachments. This is more common in myopic eyes of −6.00 D (high myopia) and most common if greater than −10.00 D (pathologic myopia).

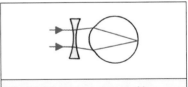

Fig. 21 Myopic eye.

Astigmatism

In this condition, which affects 85% of people, the eye is shaped like a football. Rays entering the eye are not refracted uniformly in all meridians. Regular astigmatism occurs when the corneal curvature is uniformly different in meridians at right angles to each other. It is corrected with spectacles. For example, take the case of astigmatism in the horizontal (180°) meridian (Fig. 23). A slit beam of vertical light (AB) is focused on the retina, and (CD) anterior to the retina. To correct this

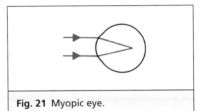

Fig. 22 Myopic eye corrected by concave lens.

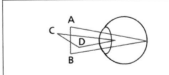

Fig. 23 Myopic astigmatism. For explanation, see text.

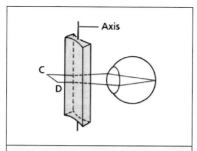

Fig. 24 Myopic astigmatism corrected with a myopic cylinder, axis 90°.

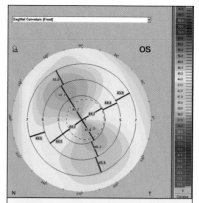

Fig. 25 Tomographic image of corneal astigmatism with the steepest power +47.70 D at axis 120° and the flattest +44.51 D at 30°. To correct this myopic astigmatic error, a −3.00 D myopic cylindrical lens would be placed in the spectacle at 30°. Courtesy of Richard Witlin, MD.

regular astigmatism, a myopic cylindrical lens (Figs 24 and 25) is used that diverges only CD.

Irregular astigmatism is caused by a distorted cornea, usually resulting from an injury or a disease called keratoconus (see Figs 40 and 264–267).

Presbyopia

This is a decrease in near vision, which occurs in all people at about age 43. The normal eye has to adjust +2.50 D to change focus from distance to near. This is called accommodation (Fig. 348). The eye's ability to accommodate decreases from +14 D at age 14 to +2 D at age 50.

Middle-aged persons are given reading glasses with plus lenses that require updating with age.

40–45 years	+1.00 to +1.50 D
50 years	+1.50 to +2.00 D
Over 55 years	+2.00 to +2.50 D

The additional plus lens in a full reading glass (Fig. 26) blurs distance vision. Half glasses (Fig. 27) and bifocals (Fig. 28) are options that allow for clear distance vision when looking up. No-line progressive bifocals are more attractive, but more expensive.

Fig. 26 Full reading glass blurs distance vision.

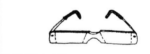

Fig. 27 Half glasses.

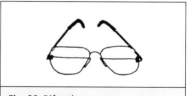

Fig. 28 Bifocals.

Refraction

Refraction is the technique of determining the lenses necessary to correct the optical defects of the eye.

Trial case and lenses

The lens case (Fig. 29) contains convex and concave spherical and cylindrical lenses. The diopter
power of spherical lenses and the axis of cylindrical lenses are recorded on the lens frames.

Trial frame

The trial frame (Fig. 30) holds the trial lenses.
Place the strongest spherical lenses in the
compartment closest to the eye because the
effective power of the lens varies with its
distance from the eye. Place the cylindrical
lenses in the compartment farthest from the
eye so that the axis can be measured on the
scale of the trial frame (0–180°).

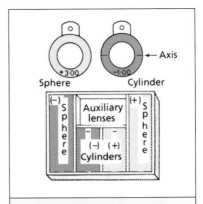

Fig. 29 Lens case with red concave and black convex lenses.

Streak retinoscopy ("flash")

This is the objective means of determining the
refractive error in all patients before beginning a subjective refraction. It is the primary
means to determine eyeglass prescriptions
in infants and illiterate persons who cannot
give adequate subjective responses. Hold the
retinoscope (Fig. 31) at arm's length from the
eye and direct its linear beam onto the pupil.
To determine the axis of astigmatism, rotate
the beam until it parallels the pupillary reflex
(Fig. 32), then move it back and forth at that
axis, as demonstrated in Fig. 33.

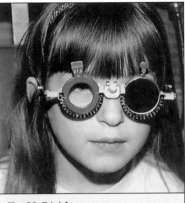

Fig. 30 Trial frame.

If the reflex moves the same way that the retinoscope beam is moving ("with motion"), a
plus (+) lens is added to the trial frame. If the
reflex moves in the opposite direction ("against
motion"), a negative (–) lens is needed. Absence
of "with motion" or "against motion" indicates the endpoint. Add –1.50 D to the above
findings to approximate the refractive error of
the meridian. Rotate the beam 90° to refract
the other axis. Computerized autorefractors
are available to perform the same task.

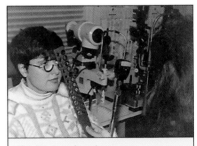

Fig. 31 Streak retinoscope.

Manifest

A manifest is the subjective trial of lenses.
Place the approximate lenses, as determined

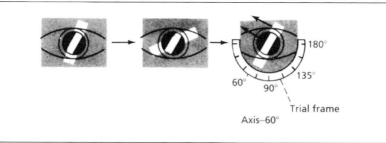

Fig. 32 Retinoscopic determination of the axis of astigmatism.

by the old spectacles or retinoscopy, in a trial frame. Occlude one of the patient's eyes, and refine the sphere by the addition of (+) and (−) 0.25 D lenses. Ask which lens makes the letter clearer. Next, refine the cylinder axis by rotating the lens in the direction of clearest vision. Test the cylinder power by adding (+) and (−) cylinders at that axis.

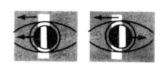

Fig. 33 Pupillary reflex with motion and against motion.

In presbyopic patients, determine the reading "add" after distance correction.

The following abbreviations are used to record the results of the refraction: W, old spectacle prescription as determined in a lensometer; F, "flash," the refractive error by retinoscopy; M, manifest, the subjective correction by trial and error; Rx, final prescription, usually equal to M.

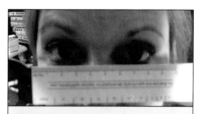

Fig. 34 Measurement of interpupillary distance.

A bifocal prescription for a farsighted presbyopic patient with astigmatism is written as shown in Fig. 36. The prescription for glasses is determined by an ophthalmologist or an optometrist. That prescription is then given to an optician who fits it into a proper frame. They measure the interpupillary distance both near and far (Fig. 34) so that the eyes' central visual axis corresponds to the optic centers of the lens. The bifocal height for the particular frame is then determined (Fig. 35).

Plastic lenses are typically prescribed because they are lighter and have less chance of shattering. This is especially important in children. Lenses are made thicker in occupational safety glasses. Glass has the advantage of being more resistant to scratching.

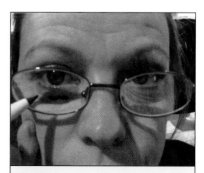

Fig. 35 Determination of bifocal segment height.

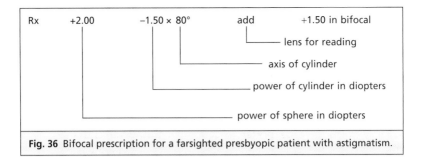

| Rx | +2.00 | −1.50 × 80° | add | +1.50 in bifocal |

lens for reading

axis of cylinder

power of cylinder in diopters

power of sphere in diopters

Fig. 36 Bifocal prescription for a farsighted presbyopic patient with astigmatism.

For photophobia, grey tints are often prescribed because they distort all colors equally. Polaroid lenses minimize glare while driving, boating, or skiing by blocking horizontal light waves. The sun's harmful ultraviolet UVA and UVB rays may cause skin cancer, photokeratitis, pinguecula (Figs 276 and 277), and pterygium (Figs 273–275), while hastening the onset of cataracts and macular degeneration. Tinted lenses, including polaroid lenses, should have a ultraviolet filter added to remove 98–100% of these rays. Branded photochromic glass lenses and Transitions plastic lenses darken in sunlight and have an ultraviolet filter.

Sports injuries, especially in basketball, baseball, ice hockey, and racket games, are a leading cause of blindness in children. Protective eye wear could prevent 90% of these sports-related injuries.

Contact lenses

Plastic contact lenses, invented in 1947, are now worn by over 40 million Americans, as an alternative to spectacles, to correct myopia, hyperopia, astigmatism, and presbyopia (Figs 37 and 38).

Other uses of contact lenses include the following:

• correction of vision in cases of an irregularly shaped cornea,
• tinted and colored lenses for cosmetic effect (see Fig. 48) and for reducing photophobia,
• prosthetic artificial eyes to cover a disfigurement or enucleated socket (Fig. 395),

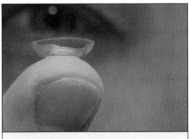

Fig. 37 Plastic contact lens.

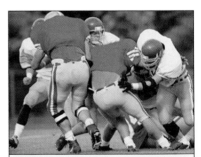

Fig. 38 Contacts are beneficial for every sport.

- bandage lenses to relieve discomfort due to blinking associated with corneal abrasions and edema.

Candidates for contact lenses

This text will discuss soft lenses because they account for 95% of fittings. Hard and gas-permeable contacts may be preferred less often for cases of dry eye, astigmatism, and irregularly shaped corneas in keratoconus (see Figs 264–267).

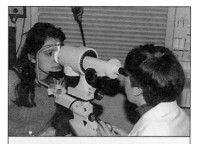

Fig. 39 Manual keratometer.

Relative contraindications to contact lens wear:
- significant allergies,
- lid margin infections (blepharitis),
- conjunctivitis,
- dry eyes,
- very young children or elderly.

Fitting contact lenses

Keratometry

After the refraction for spectacles, the corneal curvature is measured with a manual (Fig. 39) or computerized keratometer. The keratometer reveals distortion of the cornea from unhealthy contact lens wear (Fig. 40) or other corneal diseases. Power (P), base curvature (BC), and diameter (DIA) are the three basic variables that are usually required to order all types of soft lens (Figs 41–43). Curvature determines whether a flatter or steeper lens should be fitted (Fig. 43).

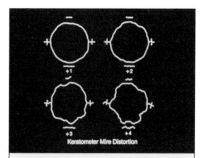

Fig. 40 Manual keratometer showing circular images projected on a damaged cornea with distorted keratometric readings.

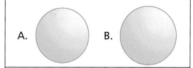

Fig. 41 (A) 13.5 mm diameter. (B) 14.5 mm diameter.

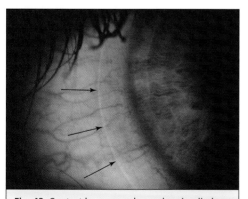

Fig. 42 Contact lens properly overlapping limbus.

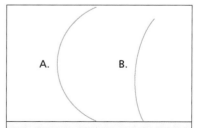

Fig. 43 (A) Steep base curve, 8.2 mm. (B) Flat base curve, 9.1 mm.

Determination of lens power

The power of a contact lens is not always the same as the patient's spectacle correction. Place a contact lens with the patient's spectacle power on the eye. Then, refine it with an over-refraction. The lens should completely cover the cornea and extend just beyond the entire limbus (corneoscleral junction; Fig. 42) and move 0.5 to 1.0 mm on each blink. If adequate centration is not achieved, a different base curve or diameter may be tried.

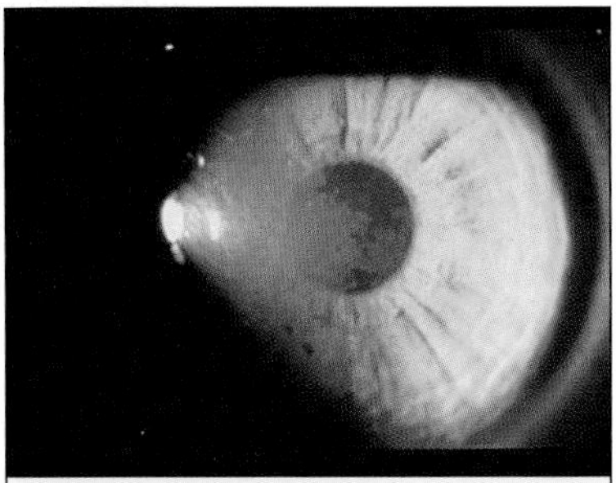

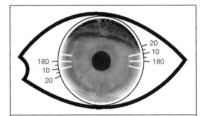

Fig. 44 Mucus deposits on contact lenses.

Types of contact lens

Most people wear contacts during the day only ("daily wear"). Sleep-in lenses ("extended wear") are used less often because they have a rate of infection that is five times as great as that for daily wear lenses. Lenses may be replaced yearly, but are more commonly disposed of every 2 weeks to 3 months ("frequent replacement") or on a daily basis ("disposable"). The frequency of replacement depends on comfort and the rate of mucus accumulation (Fig. 44).

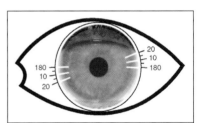

Fig. 45 Lens properly aligned on eye with center marking at 180°.

Astigmatism lenses (toric) are preferred when the astigmatism correction is −0.75 or more. They are elliptical in shape with markings on the 90° or 180° axis and are weighted at 6 o'clock so they don't rotate (Figs 45 and 46). When placed on the eye, these lines should align close to the 90° axis or a compensatory adjustment needs to be made in the prescribed lens.

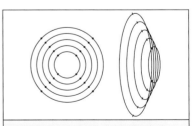

Fig. 46 Lens settled onto eye rotated 10° counterclockwise.

Presbyopic bifocal contact lenses are not highly successful, but may be tried for motivated patients – often over age 40 – who have problems focusing up close (Fig. 47). An alternative to a bifocal contact lens in correcting a presbyopic patient is to use a standard spherical contact lens, making one eye focused for near and the other focused for distance. This is called monovision. Usually, the dominant eye with the clearest vision is chosen for distance.

The iris color can be enhanced with transparent tinted soft lenses or changed to a

Fig. 47 Bifocal contact lens with concentric zones of alternating near and far vision.

different color with opaque tinted lenses (Fig. 48).

No patient should leave the office without feeling adept at lens insertion and removal, realizing the importance of good hand-washing techniques, and having knowledge about the use and differences between disinfecting, cleaning, and rinsing (saline) solutions (Figs 49–51). They also should have a backup pair of glasses.

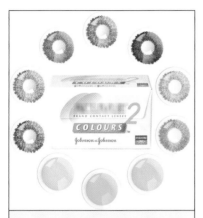

Fig. 48 Colored contact lenses.

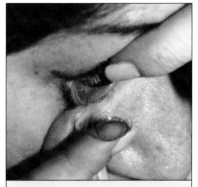

Fig. 49 Place contact lens directly on the cornea using the tip of the index finger for the contact lens, the middle finger to hold the lower lid down, and the finger of the other hand to lift the upper lid.

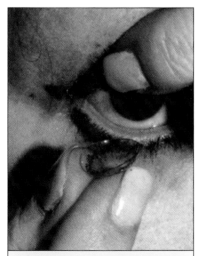

Fig. 50 Remove lens by sliding it off cornea onto sclera and then gently pinching it off using thumb and index finger.

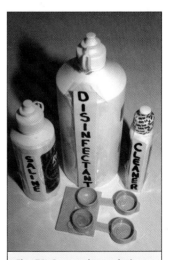

Fig. 51 Contact lens solutions.

Common problems

A 2010 study of 144,799 device-associated visits of children to emergency departments showed contact lenses to be the primary cause of adverse events (23%). Corneal abrasions, conjunctivitis, and hemorrhage were most frequent.

1 Corneal abrasions and edema are highlighted when fluorescein dye is placed in the eye and illuminated with cobalt blue light. Areas of lost or damaged corneal epithelial cells take up the dye and appear brighter (Figs 52 and 224).

2 The upper palpebral conjunctiva is the area most often irritated by contact lenses. It is called papillary conjunctivitis (Fig. 53), and is often aggravated by contact lens deposits, especially in allergic individuals. It responds well to more frequent lens replacement.

3 The bulbar conjunctiva surrounding the cornea reddens when the cornea is being compromised, as with tight-fitting lenses (Fig. 54).

4 Infected corneal ulcers (Figs 242–244) are the most serious complication and most threatening to vision.

Refractive surgery

The refractive power of the eye may be altered by surgically reshaping the cornea (Fig. 55). Radial keratotomy, invented in the Soviet Union, began in 1978 and was the most popular refractive surgery in the USA until 1996 (Fig. 56). It is hardly ever performed today. In this procedure, the cornea is

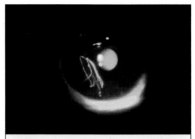

Fig. 52 Fluorescein staining of the cornea.

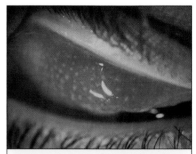

Fig. 53 Papillary conjunctivitis with characteristic redness and small, whitish elevations of conjunctiva.

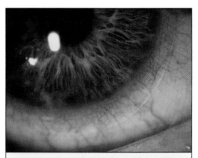

Fig. 54 Limbal injection from a tight-fitting lens.

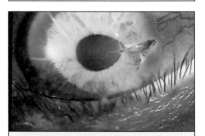

Fig. 56 Rare instance of traumatic rupture of radial keratotomy wound. Courtesy of Leo Bores.

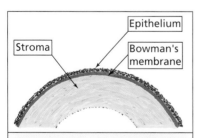

Fig. 55 Normal cornea. The average central thickness is 545 μm, about half the thickness of the peripheral cornea.

Epithelium
Stroma
Bowman's membrane

flattened with between four and eight radial incisions through 90% of the corneal depth. It has lost popularity due to slow healing, the inability to accurately predict the amount of correction, variable vision throughout the day, glare, halos, infection, and corneal perforation with secondary cataract formation.

Three newer procedures – LASIK, PRK, and epi-LASIK – correct myopia, hyperopia, and astigmatism by utilizing an excimer laser to remove corneal stroma. In order for the laser to effectively reach the stroma, the corneal epithelium must be gotten out of the way. The three techniques vary in the way this is accomplished.

1 Laser in situ keratomileusis (LASIK) (Figs 57–61) is the most frequently performed cosmetic surgery in the USA. Many millions of procedures have been done since its introduction in 1990. A flap of epithelium, Bowman's membrane, and stroma is created with a blade or femtosecond laser. Then a different laser, called an excimer, is used to ablate and thin the underlying stromal bed.

A disadvantage of LASIK is a resulting decrease in ocular rigidity. This is due to loss of ablated stromal bed and decreased effectiveness of stroma remaining in the flap since it never

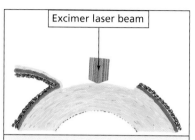

Excimer laser beam

Fig. 57 LASIK: a 110 μm flap of epithelium, Bowman's membrane, and stroma is created with a blade or laser. Then, an excimer laser ablates the stroma. The post-LASIK stromal bed should be at least 250 μm to prevent ectasia.

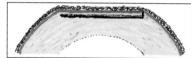

Fig. 58 Sculpted cornea after LASIK with remaining Bowman's membrane.

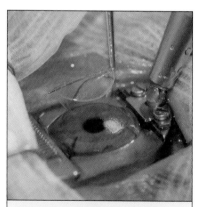

Fig. 59 Superficial corneal flap created with a microkeratome. Laser creation of flap is reported to be superior. Courtesy of Chris Barry, M.Med.Sci., and *J. Ophthalmic Photogr.*, 1999, Vol. 22, No. 1A.

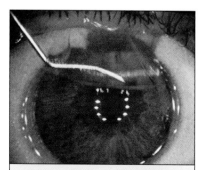

Fig. 60 LASIK surgery showing flap being lifted with spatula and laser beam on central cornea ablating stroma.

completely heals. To minimize the loss of effective stroma, the goal has been to make the thinnest possible flap (Fig. 57). Eyes with over 8 D of myopia requires a lot of stromal ablation. This thinning becomes excessive and could weaken the wall of the eye resulting an ectasia (bulging) of the cornea. The average corneal thickness is 545 µm (Fig. 55). Ectasia occurs most often with pre-op corneas thinner than 521 µm and a post-op stromal bed of less than 256 µm.

LASIK damages corneal nerve fibers, which results in the commonly occurring dry eye. Another flap complication is that corneal epithelial cells can grow under the flap and may have to be removed (Fig. 63). This occurs in about 1% of primary surgeries, but in up to 23% of cases when the flap has to be lifted for a second LASIK procedure. The flap adheres poorly and can be lifted up to 6 years after its creation, but the risk of complications from lifting the original flap for retreatment incrementally increases after 1 year. Trauma may dislocate this flap for many years after its creation (Fig. 62).

2 An alternative to LASIK is photorefractive keratectomy (PRK) (Figs 64–66). It eliminates a need for a flap by mechanically creating a central corneal abrasion to remove the epithelium (Fig. 64). The advantage is it leaves more functioning stroma. The disadvantage is pain from the abrasion and slower return of vision.

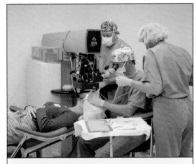

Fig. 61 Excimer laser used to remove a layer of central corneal stroma.

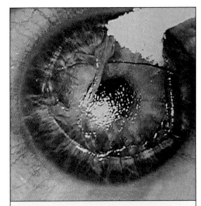

Fig. 62 Late dislocation of a LASIK flap by self-inflicted injury. Courtesy of C.K. Patel, BSC, FRC Ophth., and *Arch. Ophthalmol.*, Mar. 2001, Vol. 119, p. 447. Copyright 2001, American Medical Association.

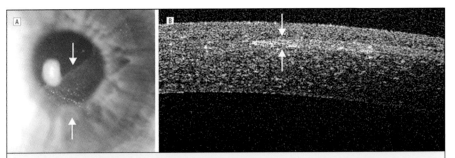

Fig. 63 (A) Grey area (arrows) where epithelial cells grew under the flap. (B) OCT scan showing cells. If cells are near the central cornea, or if there is overlying melting in the peripheral cornea, the flap must be lifted and cells removed. Courtesy of V. Charistopoulos, MD, and *Arch. Ophthalmol.*, Aug. 2007, Vol. 125, pp. 1027–1036. Copyright 2007, American Medical Association.

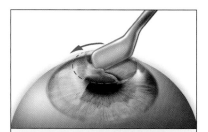

Fig. 64 Removal of corneal epithelium precedes excimer laser thinning of cornea in PRK.

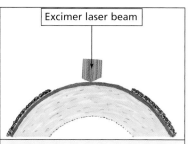

Excimer laser beam

Fig. 65 PRK laser ablation of Bowman's membrane and stroma after mechanical debridement of epithelium.

3 The newest technique, called epi-LASIK (Fig. 67) creates an epithelial flap that includes no stroma. As a consequence, there will be more stroma remaining to contribute to ocular rigidity. However, the epithelial flap heals more slowly than the LASIK flap so that vision takes longer to recover. It heals faster and causes less pain than PRK, in which there is a total corneal abrasion after surgery.

All three laser techniques usually yield good results, but may be complicated by infection, glare, halos, dry eye, over- or under-correction of refractive error, and unknown long-term effects. LASIK has been by far the most popular corneal refractive surgery for the past two decades with about 1 million procedures per year. A recent survey revealed slightly over half of ophthalmologists would consider laser refractive surgery on themselves.

Intracorneal ring segment implants are a less frequently used alternative to flattening the cornea. They correct small amounts of myopia and keratoconus. The procedure involves the placement of a plastic ring with arc lengths of 90–355° in the peripheral cornea (Fig. 68). Proponents argue that unlike LASIK, it is safer because it doesn't involve surgery on the central visual axis.

Large amounts of hyperopia (over 4 D) and myopia (over 8 D) are difficult to correct with reshaping the cornea because it becomes too thin and unstable. Intraocular lenses can be inserted inside the eye (Fig. 69) to correct these larger refractive errors, but have all the inherent risks associated with intraocular

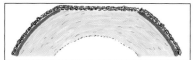

Fig. 66 Sculpted cornea after PRK or epi-LASIK.

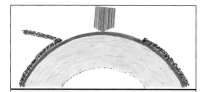

Fig. 67 Epi-LASIK: creation of epithelial flap with blade followed by laser ablation of stroma.

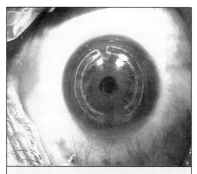

Fig. 68 Intracorneal ring segment. Courtesy of Dimitri Azar, MD.

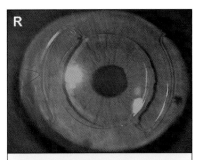

Fig. 69 Phakic 6H2 anterior chamber intraocular lens to correct refractive errors. Courtesy of Oil, Inc.

surgery. There has to be a safe space between the implanted lens, the cornea, and the patient's natural lens or corneal edema and/or cataract could occur.

A technique called corneal limbal relaxing incisions may be used to correct astigmatism. A manual (blade) or femtosecond laser creates an arcurate incision to a depth of 600 μm (80% of corneal thickness) on the steepest corneal meridian. It is usually used to correct 0.75 to 2.00 D of astigmatism (Figs 70–72). The amount of correction is determined by whether one or two incisions are used and by the depth and length of each, which may vary from 2 to 3 clock hours.

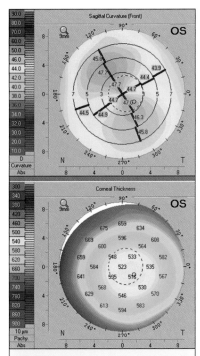

Fig. 70 Tomograms of corneal topography measure 25,000 points of elevation in 5 seconds, giving the dioptic power of the anterior and posterior cornea and corneal thickness. Courtesy of Richard Witlin, MD.

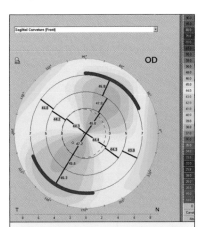

Fig. 71 Limbal relaxing incision at 60° (the steepest meridian) super-imposed (in red) on a tomographic image. It corrects negative astigmatism at 150°. Courtesy of Richard Witlin, MD.

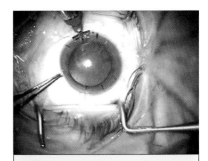

Fig. 72 Manual limbal relaxing incison being created on steepest axis at 100° to correct negative astigmatism at 10°. Courtesy of Bonnie Henderson, Harvard Medical School.

Chapter 3
Neuro-ophthalmology

Six muscles move each eye around three axes. They are innervated by the III, IV, and VI cranial nerves.

Eye movements

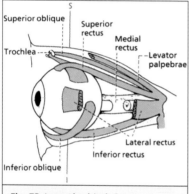

Fig. 73 Lateral orbital view: adduction and abduction are around the superior–inferior axis (SI).

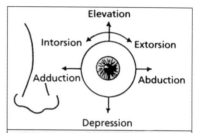

Fig. 74 The eye rotates around three different axes coordinated by the action of six extraocular muscles.

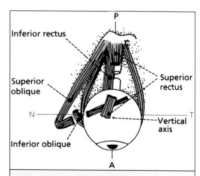

Fig. 75 Superior orbital view. Elevation and depression are on the horizontal axis (NT, nasal–temporal) passing from the nasal to temporal side of the eye. Torsion is on the anterior–posterior axis (AP).

Manual for Eye Examination and Diagnosis, Ninth edition. Mark Leitman.
© 2017 John Wiley & Sons, Inc. Published 2017 by John Wiley & Sons, Inc.

Six extraocular muscles that rotate the eye

Muscle	Actions	Neural control
Medial rectus	Adducts	Oculomotor nerve (CN III)
Inferior rectus	Mainly depresses, also extorts, adducts	Oculomotor nerve (CN III)
Superior rectus	Mainly elevates, also intorts, adducts	Oculomotor nerve (CN III)
Inferior oblique	Mainly extorts, also elevates, abducts	Oculomotor nerve (CN III)
Superior oblique	Mainly intorts, also depresses, abducts	Trochlear nerve (CN IV)
Lateral rectus	Abducts	Abducens nerve (CN VI)

CN, cranial nerve.

Nerves to ocular structures

Optic nerve Cranial nerve (CN) II	The axon of the retinal ganglion cell which transmits visual impulse from the eye to the brain	
Oculomotor nerve (CN III)	Innervates	Action
Motor (1–5)	1 Medial rectus muscle	Adducts
	2 Inferior rectus muscle	Mainly depresses, also extorts, adducts
	3 Superior rectus muscle	Mainly elevates, also intorts, adducts
	4 Inferior oblique muscle	Mainly extorts, also elevates, abducts
	5 Levator palpebrae muscle	Elevates upper lid
Parasympathetic (6 and 7)	6 Pupil constrictor muscle	Responds to light and near focus
	7 Ciliary muscle	Focuses lens for near
Trochlear nerve (CN IV)	Superior oblique muscle	Mainly intorts, also depresses, abducts
Trigeminal nerve	CN V1: eye, upper lid, orbit, and nose CN V2: lower lid	Sensory
Abducens nerve (CN VI)	Lateral rectus muscle	Abducts
Facial nerve (CN VII)	Orbicularis muscle	Closes upper and lower lids
Sympathetic nerve	1 Müller's muscle	1 Elevates upper lid
	2 Pupil dilator muscle	2 Opens pupil in response to stress, "fight or flight," and adrenergic drugs
	3 Skin of lid	3 Sweat glands

CN, cranial nerve.

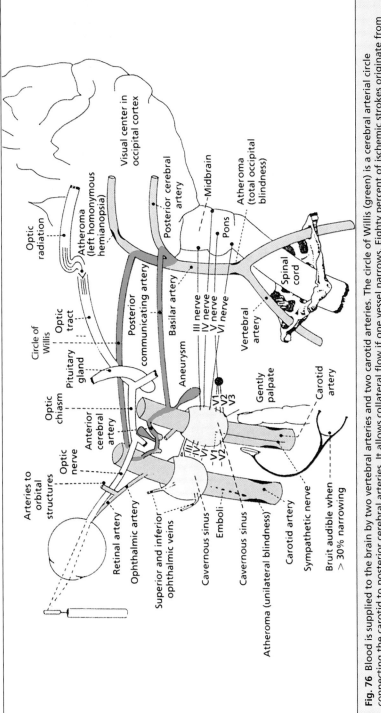

Fig. 76 Blood is supplied to the brain by two vertebral arteries and two carotid arteries. The circle of Willis (green) is a cerebral arterial circle connecting the carotid to posterior cerebral arteries. It allows collateral flow if one vessel narrows. Eighty percent of ischemic strokes originate from the carotid and 20% from the vertebral or basilar circulation. The two most common cerebral aneurysms occur in this circle. The one connecting the two anterior cerebral arteries may press on the optic chiasm, sometimes causing a bitemporal hemianopsia. The other, at the junction of the carotid and posterior communicating arteries, may press on CN III, causing a dilated pupil. If the aneurysms rupture, they may cause a severe headache, stiff painful neck, blurred or double vision, and photophobia.

Labels in figure:

- Visual center in occipital cortex
- Optic radiation
- Atheroma (left homonymous hemianopsia)
- Posterior cerebral artery
- Midbrain
- Atheroma (total occipital blindness)
- Pons
- Basilar artery
- Posterior communicating artery
- Spinal cord
- III nerve
- IV nerve
- V nerve
- VI nerve
- Vertebral artery
- Circle of Willis
- Optic tract
- Pituitary gland
- Aneurysm
- V1
- V2
- V3
- Gently palpate
- Carotid artery
- Optic chiasm
- Anterior cerebral artery
- Optic nerve
- III
- IV
- VI
- V1
- V2
- Arteries to orbital structures
- Retinal artery
- Ophthalmic artery
- Superior and inferior ophthalmic veins
- Cavernous sinus
- Emboli
- Cavernous sinus
- Atheroma (unilateral blindness)
- Carotid artery
- Sympathetic nerve
- Bruit audible when > 30% narrowing

Strabismus

Strabismus refers to the nonalignment of the eyes such that an object in space is not visualized simultaneously by the fovea of each eye.

If one eye is occluded while both eyes are fusing, the occluded eye may turn in (esophoria, noted with the letter E) or out (exophoria, X). Small phorias are usually asymptomatic. A phoria may degenerate into a tropia. A tropia is an eyeturn that occurs spontaneously. A tropia is more likely to occur as the amount of the phoria increases and as the patient's ability to compensate decreases. This occurs with tiredness later in the day and from any stimulus that dissociates the eyes, such as poor vision in one eye. Absence of a phoria (perfectly straight eyes) is termed orthophoria.

Complications of strabismus

Amblyopia

Also called lazy eye, amblyopia is decreased vision due to improper use of an eye in childhood. The two common causes are an eyeturn (strabismic amblyopia) or a refractive error (refractive amblyopia), uncorrected before age 8. In strabismus, children unconsciously suppress the deviated eye to avoid diplopia.

Types of tropia	
Esotropia (ET)	Deviation of eye nasally
Exotropia (XT)	Deviation of eye outward (temporally)
Hypertropia (HT)	Deviation of eye upward
Intermittent tropia	A phoria that spontaneously breaks to a tropia; indicate with parentheses. Example: R (ET) = right intermittent esotropia.
Constant monocular tropia	Present at all times in one eye. Example: RXT, constant right exotropia. Often associated with loss of vision, if onset is in childhood.
Alternating tropia	Either eye can deviate. Vision is usually equal in both eyes.

Strabismic amblyopia is treated by patching the good eye (Fig. 77), thereby forcing the child to use the amblyopic eye. The better eye is patched full time: 1 week for each year of age. It is repeated until there is no improvement on two consecutive visits.

Refractive amblyopia is treated by correcting the refractive error with glasses and patching the better eye. Both types must be treated in early childhood because after age 5 it is difficult to improve vision. After age 8, improvement is almost impossible, but should be tried.

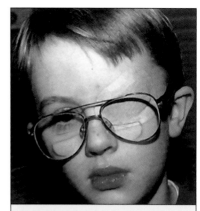
Fig. 77 Patching for amblyopia.

Poor cosmetic appearance

Tropias that cannot be corrected with spectacles may be cosmetically unacceptable and the patient may desire surgery.

Loss of fusion

Fusion occurs when the images from both eyes are perceived as one object, with resulting stereopsis (three-dimensional vision). Many patients with tropias never gain the ability to fuse. Finer grades of fusion are assessed by using the Wirt stereopsis test (see Fig. 78).

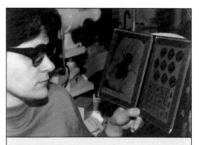
Fig. 78 Wirt stereopsis.

Wirt stereopsis test (Fig. 78)

While wearing polarized glasses, the patient views a test card. The degree of fusion is determined by the number of pictures correctly described in three dimensions.

Near point of convergence (NPC) (Fig. 79)

The NPC is the closest point at which the eyes can cross to view a near object. It is measured by having the patient make a maximal effort to fixate on a small object as it is moved toward his or her eyes. The distance at which the eyes stop converging and one turns out is recorded as the NPC. Convergence insufficiency must be considered if the NPC is greater than 8 cm. These patients may complain of

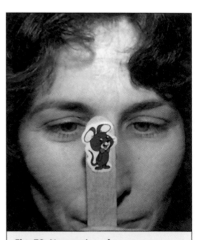
Fig. 79 Near point of convergence.

diplopia or other difficulties while reading. Exercises or prism glasses may help.

Accommodative esotropia (Figs 80 and 81)

When the lens of a normal eye focuses, it simultaneously causes the eyes to converge. Patients with hyperopia who are not wearing glasses must focus the lens of their eye (accommodation) to see clearly near and far. This focusing stimulates the accommodative reflex, causing convergence of the eyes. When the ratio of convergence to accommodation is abnormally high, an esotropia results, which corrects with lenses.

Nonaccommodative esotropia
(Figs 82–84)

This is due to a defect in the brain not related to the accommodative reflex. It is corrected by surgically weakening the medial rectus muscle by recessing its insertion posteriorly on the sclera or by tightening the lateral rectus muscle by resecting part of it. Less often, botulinum toxin is injected to weaken eye muscles.

An epicanthal skin fold connects the nasal upper and lower lids (Fig. 85) and is common in infants and Asians. It gives the false impression of a cross-eye, called pseudostrabismus.

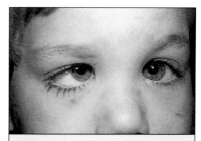

Fig. 80 Accommodative esotropia.

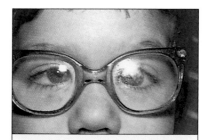

Fig. 81 Accommodative esotropia corrected with hyperopic lenses.

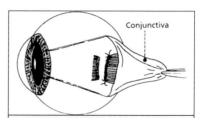

Fig. 82 Recession to weaken muscle.

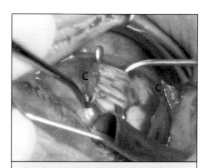

Fig. 84 Strabismus surgery: after incising the conjunctiva (C), the medial rectus muscle is exposed and isolated with two muscle hooks. Courtesy of Elliot Davidoff, MD.

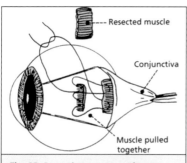

Fig. 83 Resection to strengthen muscle.

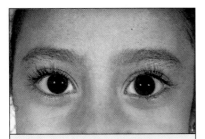

Fig. 85 Epicanthal folds causing a false impression of cross-eye (pseudostrabismus).

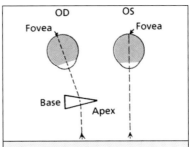

Fig. 86 Right esotropia neutralized with prism (apex-in).

Measurement of the amount of eye-turn with prisms

Ocular deviations are measured in prism diopters. When light passes through a prism, it is bent toward the base of the prism. One prism diopter (1 Δ) displaces the image 1 cm at a distance of 1 m from the prism. Do not confuse prism diopters (Δ) with lens diopters (D).

In a right esotropia, the right fovea is turned temporally. To focus the light on the right fovea, a prism (apex-in) is placed in front of the right eye (Fig. 86). For an exotropia, use apex-out. *Rule:* point the prism apex in the direction of the tropia.

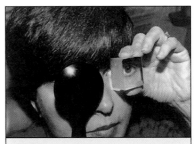

Fig. 87 Prism cover test.

Prism cover test for measurement of eye-turn (Fig. 87)

The patient fixates on an object at 20 ft (6 m). When the fixating eye is occluded, the deviated eye must move to look at the target. Increasing amounts of prism are placed in front of the deviated eye until no movement is noted when the cover is moved back and forth over each eye.

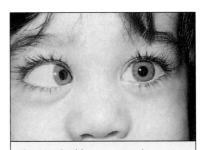

Fig. 88 Hirschberg: esotropia.

Hirschberg's test

When the cover test is difficult to perform on young children, the angle of strabismus can be estimated by using Hirschberg's test (Figs 88–90). As the child fixates on a point source of light, the position of the corneal light reflex is noted. Each 1 mm of deviation

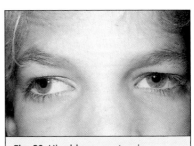

Fig. 89 Hirschberg: exotropia.

from the center of the cornea is equivalent to approximately 14 Δ of deviation. A reflex 2 mm temporal to the center of the cornea indicates an esotropia of approximately 28 Δ.

Causes of strabismus

1 Paralytic strabismus is due to cranial nerve (III, IV, or VI) disease or eye-muscle weakness from thyroid disease, traumatic contusions, myasthenia gravis, or orbital floor fractures.
2 Nonparalytic strabismus is due to a malfunction of a center in the brain. It is often inherited and begins in childhood.

Demonstration of paralytic strabismus

In paralytic strabismus, the amount of deviation is greatest when gaze is directed in the field of action of the weakened muscle. To demonstrate underaction of any of the 12 external ocular muscles, the patient fixates on an object moved into each of the six cardinal fields of gaze (Fig. 91). Each position

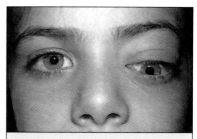

Fig. 90 Hirschberg: left hypotropia.

Comparison of paralytic and nonparalytic strabismus

	Paralytic	Nonparalytic
Age of onset	Usually in older persons	Usually starts before 6 years of age
Complaint since	Diplopia	Cosmetic eye-turn; less diplopia: child suppresses deviated eye
Eye-turn	Largest deviation in field of action of affected muscle	No one muscle is underactive; deviation similar in all directions
Vision	Not affected	Deviated eye may have loss of vision (amblyopia)
Plan	Neurologic workup	Ophthalmic workup

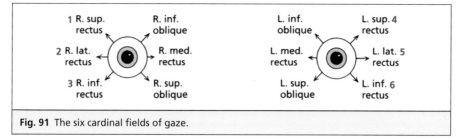

Fig. 91 The six cardinal fields of gaze.

tests one muscle of each eye (e.g., position 3 tests the right inferior rectus and the left superior oblique muscles). In addition to observing for underaction or overaction of the muscles, ask the patient where diplopia is greatest. For exact measurements, use the prism cover test.

Most often the cause for cranial nerve (CN) III, IV, and VI paralysis cannot be confirmed, since it is due to ischemia from small-vessel closure. In adults, ischemia from diabetes is the most common cause and often resolves within 10 weeks. Testing is done to rule out causes such as multiple sclerosis, aneurysms, neoplasms, and other rarer conditions, especially in younger individuals where vessel closure is not likely.

Cranial nerves III–VIII

Oculomotor nerve (CN III)

CN III paralysis (Figs 92–94) results in underaction of the inferior oblique and medial, inferior, and superior rectus muscles, resulting in an eye turned down and out. Since this nerve also innervates the levator palpebral muscle, which elevates the lid and the pupillary constrictor muscle, the lid is drooped and the pupil is dilated. CN III paralysis due to diabetes often spares the pupil.

Always examine for a dilated pupil after head trauma. CN III parallels the posterior communicating artery (see Figs 76, 95, 96, and 136) so that ruptured aneurysms in the circle of Willis are a common cause of paralysis with a dilated pupil and an explosive headache (Figs 95 and 96). Also, CN III passes under the tentorial ridge in the brain and is highly susceptible to uncal herniation of the brain. Herniation may follow increased intracranial pressure from cerebral edema, hematoma, tumor, abscess, or cerebral spinal fluid obstruction. Although a dilated pupil is a more common ominous sign after head injury, small or unequal pupils could indicate serious insults to other parts of the brain.

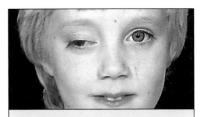

Fig. 92 Right CN III paralysis. In straight gaze, eye turns down and out with dilated pupil and ptosis.

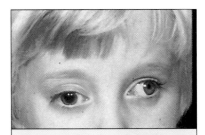

Fig. 93 Inability of right eye to look to the left due to medial rectus paralysis.

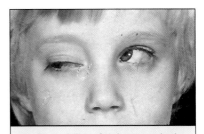

Fig. 94 Inability of right eye to look up to right due to superior rectus paralysis. Courtesy of David Taylor.

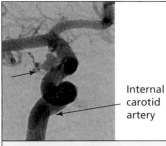

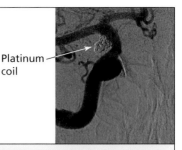

Platinum coil

Fig. 95 Cerebral angiogram of right carotid artery showing a 3 mm × 4 mm posterior communicating arterial aneurysm (↑). This occurred in a 50 year-old man with a subarachnoid hemorrhage and the worst headache of his life. Fifteen percent of patients with subarachnoid hemorrhages die before reaching the hospital. Aneurysms may be surgically clipped or obliterated with endovascular coiling.

Fig. 96 Stent-assisted platinum coiling embolization of aneurysm. A small electric charge is sent to the linear platinum tip when it enters the aneurysm. This charge detaches it, causes folding, and promotes thrombosis. Courtesy of Stavropoula I. Tjoumakaris, MD, and Robert Rosenwasser, MD, Thomas Jefferson University Hospital Endovascular Neurological Surgery Department.

Trochlear nerve (CN IV)

The trochlear nerve (CN IV) innervates the superior oblique muscle. Since this muscle acts as a depressor when the eye is rotated nasally, its paralysis causes patients to have diplopia when looking down to read. Since intorsion is this muscle's main action, there is a head tilt to the opposite shoulder so that the eye doesn't have to be intorted (Fig. 97). If the doctor forces the patient's head straight (Fig. 98), the superior rectus must act as an intorter. Since the superior rectus also elevates the eye as it intorts, vertical diplopia occurs. A common cause of superior oblique muscle dysfunction is trauma since it passes through the trochlea (see Fig. 73), where it is accessible to injury due to its location just under the superior nasal orbital rim. All patients with a head tilt should be checked for trochlear nerve dysfunction.

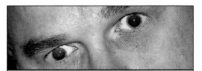

Fig. 97 Left superior oblique paralysis. To avoid diplopia, head is tilted to the opposite shoulder. Courtesy of Joseph Calhoun.

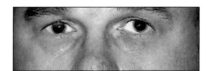

Fig. 98 Paralytic left superior oblique with vertical diplopia in primary gaze. Note: sclera visible below left cornea.

Abducens nerve (CN VI)

The abducens nerve (CN VI) innervates the lateral rectus muscle that abducts the eye. Loss of function causes diplopia and a cross-eye (Figs 99–101). As this nerve may be damaged from increased intracranial pressure, one should be alert to an associated headache, nausea, and papilledema.

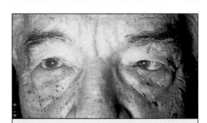

Fig. 99 Right lateral rectus paralysis in right gaze. Courtesy of Elliot Davidoff.

Trigeminal nerve (CN V)

The trigeminal nerve (CN V) is the sensory nerve of the head and face (Fig. 102).

V1   Ophthalmic branch: sensory to upper lid, eye, and nose.

V2   Maxillary branch: sensory to lower lid and cheek.

V3   Mandibular branch: no ocular action.

Injury may cause an anesthetic effect, as occurs in an orbital blow-out fracture (Figs 216–218), or pain, as occurs in herpes zoster dermatitis (shingles; Fig. 103) and trigeminal neuralgia (tic douloureux).

Herpes zoster dermatitis affects 1 in 3 people in the USA, especially the elderly. It is due to reactivation of the latent varicella virus introduced during an episode of chicken pox in childhood. It often affects the ophthalmic division of CN V. There may be associated iritis, keratitis, a fever, and adenopathy. Rx: valacyclovir (Valtrex)

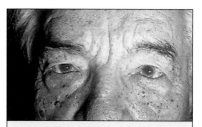

Fig. 100 Right lateral rectus paralysis, straight gaze.

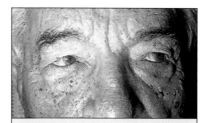

Fig. 101 Right lateral rectus paralysis left gaze.

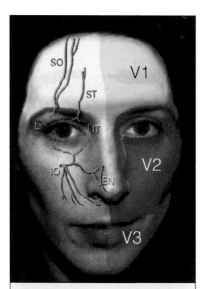

Fig. 102 The three divisions of the trigeminal nerve, V1, V2, V3, and the individual nerves. SO, supraorbital; ST, supratrochlear; L, lacrimal; IT, intratrochlear; IO, infraorbital; EN, external nasal.

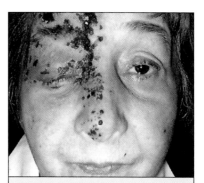

Fig. 103 Herpes zoster dermatitis. Think of shingles when the dermatitis follows the distribution of CN V and doesn't cross the facial midline.

1000 mg PO TID × 7 days. It ideally should be started within 72 hours of onset of skin lesions. The treatment for iritis is similar to the treatment for other causes for iritis. Post-herpetic neuralgia is the most common sequela. A vaccination, which reduces the incidence and severity of symptoms, is recommended for those over age 50, but is most important in the elderly and immunocompromised.

Facial nerve (CN VII)

The facial nerve (CN VII) innervates the orbicularis oculi muscle, which closes the lid, and also the muscles that control facial expression (Fig. 104). It also stimulates lacrimal secretion. The common CN VII paralysis in adults is called Bell's palsy and is usually due to ischemia or a virus (Figs 105 and 106).

Myokymia refers to minor eyelid spasms of the orbicularis muscle, which the patient senses as a twitching of the muscles of the lid and lasting for seconds or minutes. It usually goes unnoticed by an observer. It may be related to stress, fatigue, caffeine, or hyperthyroidism. Episodes may last for weeks.

Blepharospasm (Fig. 107) is a more severe spasm of the orbicularis muscle causing the eyelids to close involuntarily. The first-line treatment is to give six injections of botulinum toxin (Botox) into the muscles around the eye every 3–4 months. It blocks the release of acetylcholine at the neuromuscular junction. Severe cases may require surgical removal of muscle fibers or branches of the seventh nerve.

Vestibulocochlear nerve (CN VIII)

The vestibulocochlear nerve (CN VIII) is the sensory nerve for hearing and balance. The vestibular branch has sensory fibers in the semicircular canals and the vestibule of the inner ear. Their axons connect in a complex system to the nuclei of CN III, IV, and VI in the brainstem, which control the muscles that move the eye. This vesibulo-ocular reflex maintains fixation and balance when the head moves.

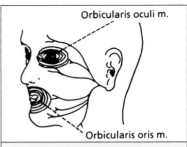

Fig. 104 Facial nerve to orbicularis oculi and oris muscles.

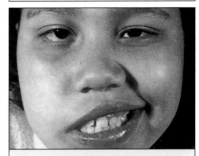

Fig. 105 Bell's palsy due to right CN VII paralysis causes incomplete blink reflex and inability to close lids completely.

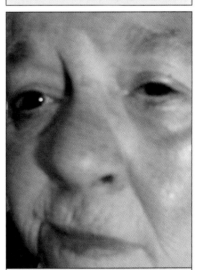

Fig. 106 In CN VII paralysis, the inability to close the eye may cause corneal dessication. To partially remedy this, the left lateral upper and lower tarsus were sutured together (tarsorrhaphy). It may be temporary or permanent.

Diseases of this pathway cause nystagmus and the illusionary whirling sensation called vertigo. The cochlear division of this nerve is responsible for hearing.

Nystagmus

Normal nystagmus

This is an involuntary rhythmic movement of the eyes in a horizontal, vertical, or rotary fashion. Pendular nystagmus means equal motion in each direction, while the jerky type has a quicker movement in one direction than the other. Fine movements are most easily seen by observing the eye with an ophthalmoscope or slit lamp.

Vestibular nystagmus is due to stimulation of the semicircular canals of the ear, either by rotating the body or placing cold or hot water in the ear.

Optokinetic nystagmus is a jerky type of movement, as occurs when one watches scenery go by while riding in a car (Fig. 108). Endpoint nystagmus is a jerky type occurring in extreme positions of gaze.

Abnormal nystagmus

Diseases of the vestibular system, originating in the inner ear or in the cerebellum, are the most common reasons for vertigo with associated nystagmus. A clue in differentiating the cause of the vertigo and nystagmus is that CN VIII disease often has signs localizing it to the ear. Cerebellar disease often has impairment of speech and gait.

Gaze nystagmus occurs in certain fields of gaze. It is caused by drugs such as Dilantin or barbiturates, demyelinating diseases, cerebral vascular insufficiency, and brain tumors. Infantile nystagmus syndrome has a pendular nystagmus starting within the first 6 months of life. It may be associated with albinism, retinal disease, or other causes of reduced vision or blindness. If there is a position of gaze

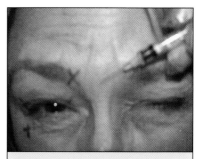

Fig. 107 Botox is injected (X) into the orbicularis oculi muscle to treat blepharospasm. Care is taken not to inject the center of the upper lid, which could paralyze the belly of the levator m., resulting in ptosis.

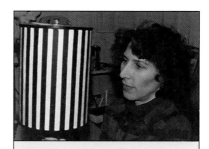

Fig. 108 Optokinetic drum that causes optokinetic nystagmus when rotated. Hysterics and malingerers faking total blindness cannot help but move their eyes.

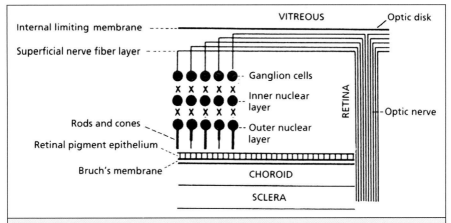

Fig. 109 Schematic cross-section of the retina. The ganglion cell fibers on the surface of the retina become covered with a myelin sheath at the optic disk and the continuation of these fibers outside the eye is then called the optic nerve.

with less movement (null angle), eye-muscle surgery or prisms may be tried to move this position to a straight-ahead gaze.

Spasmus nutans is a unilateral or bilateral pendular nystagmus beginning at about 6 months of age and often ending by 2 years of age. It may be associated with head nodding.

Optic nerve (CN II)

The optic nerve (CN II) is made up of 1.2 million retinal ganglion cell axons which transmit the visual message from the eye to the brain. The nerve begins at the optic disk (papilla) as the ganglion cell axons exit the eye (Figs 109 and 311–317). Each fiber picks up a myelin sheath as it exits the eye (Fig. 436) and the whole nerve is covered with a meningeal sheath (pia mater, arachnoid mater, and dura mater) (Fig. 118).

When the intraocular ganglion cells or the extraocular optic nerve are damaged, the normal pink or orange optic disk may turn chalk white (Fig. 110).

In the case of glaucoma, the pallor is associated with excavation (cupping) of the disk (Fig. 111).

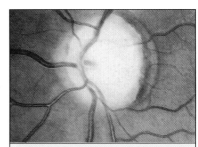

Fig. 110 Optic atrophy resulting from ischemia, transection, toxicity, or inflammation.

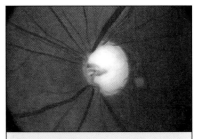

Fig. 111 Optic atrophy with cupping due to glaucoma.

Intraocular causes for loss of optic nerve fibers

Glaucoma is a disease of the optic nerve aggravated by high intraocular pressure. It is the most common cause of optic neuropathy. Therefore, a whole section is devoted to it (see Chapter 6, p. 97).

Retinal ischemia due to retinal artery and vein occlusion or diabetic closure of capillaries may cause loss of ganglion cells and result in pallor of the disk. Thinning of the ganglion cell layer also occurs in pathologic myopia, retinitis pigmentosa, chorioretinitis, and numerous less common retinal diseases.

Extraocular causes for loss of optic nerve fibers

When the nerve near the optic disk is inflamed (optic neuritis), you may see papillitis with an ophthalmoscope. Signs of papillitis include flame hemorrhages around the disk, cells in the overlying vitreous, and a blurred disk margin (Fig. 112). Optic neuritis could cause dimming of vision, reduced central vision, decreased pupil reaction to light, reduced color vision, and pain with eye movement.

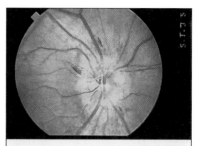

Fig. 112 Optic neuritis with papillitis.

When light is shined in a normal eye, both pupils constrict. This is called a consensual light reflex. Damage to the optic nerve (CN II) reduces direct pupillary constriction to light. The diseased eye will constrict well when light shines on the other eye due to the normal consensual reflex. Shining a light back and forth between eyes, called the swinging light test (Fig. 113), reveals the eye with optic disease to be dilating as the light shines on it due to the stronger consensual reflex wearing off. This is called a Marcus Gunn pupil and is helpful in diagnosing optic neuritis. Also, in optic neuritis, the patient claims the light is dimmer in the diseased eye as it is shined back and forth.

Fifty percent of cases of optic neuritis are due to multiple sclerosis. Multiple sclerosis is a chronic relapsing condition with a usual onset between the third and fifth decades. It has a

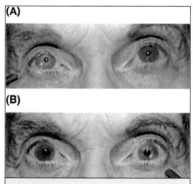

Fig. 113 Swinging light test. (A) Both pupils constrict when light shines in normal right eye due to consensual reflex. (B) Left pupil in eye with optic neuritis dilates as light shines on it, since consensual stimulation wears off.

partial autoimmune etiology that causes multiple areas of demyelination in the central nervous system (Fig. 114). Diplopia due to CN III, IV, or VI paralysis or decreased vision is often the first symptom of the disease. In multiple sclerosis, optic neuritis often occurs without papillitis. The more posterior involvement of the nerve causes more pain on eye movement due to pain fibers in the meningeal sheath covering the nerve. Corticosteroids may shorten the length of time the optic neuritis lasts, but has little effect on the final loss of vision.

The next most common cause of optic neuritis is non-inflammatory (nonarteritic) ischemia due to arteriosclerosis. This commonly occurs in older patients and there is no firmly established treatment. In this elderly population, ischemia could have an inflammatory cause and one must always consider the possibility of giant cell arteritis (GCA), also called temporal or cranial arteritis. Failure to recognize GCA early could result in bilateral blindness and even death. GCA almost always occurs after age 50 and the occurrence rises dramatically with each decade. Besides having symptoms typical of optic neuropathy, patients may also have scalp tenderness, pain on chewing, arthritis, weight loss, loss of appetite, and malaise. An elevated erythrocyte sedimentation rate and C-reactive protein with a positive temporal artery biopsy confirms the diagnosis (Figs 115–117). Prompt treatment with

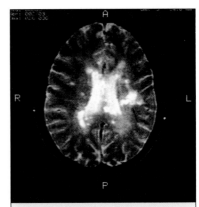

Fig. 114 Magnetic resonance imaging (MRI) of the brain. White areas of high intensity correspond to demyelinating plaques, which are present in 90% of known multiple sclerosis cases. MRI of orbit could show thickening of an inflamed optic nerve.

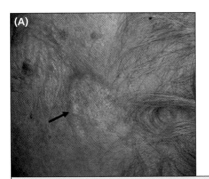
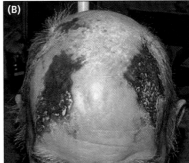

Fig. 115 Two of the clinical manifestations of cranial arteritis. (A) Photograph of an enlarged and nodular left temporal artery that is tender to palpation and pulseless. (B) Hemorrhagic necrosis of the scalp in a patient with giant cell arteritis (GCA). *Source*: Campbell et al. *Clin. Experiments Dermatol.*, 2003, Vol. 28, pp. 488–490. Reproduced with permission of Wiley.

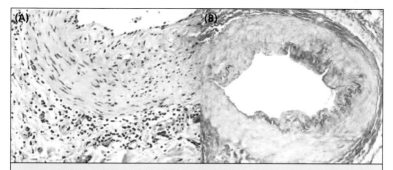

Fig. 116 Histopathologic examination of a temporal artery biopsy in a patient with giant cell arteritis (GCA). (A) Haematoxylin and eosin stain shows lymphocytic infiltration of the adventitia. (B) Elastic tissue stain shows fragmentation of the internal elastic lamina and intimal hyperplasia.

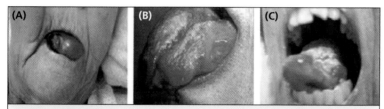

Fig. 117 Three examples of ischemic oral lesions caused by giant cell arteritis (GCA). (A) Patient with tongue and lip infarction. (B) Cyanosis and edema in the tongue. (C) A necrotic lesion of the tongue. *Source*: M. Goicochea, J. Correale, L. Bonamico et al., *Headache*, 2007, Vol. 47, pp. 1213–1215. Reproduced with permission of Wiley.

high doses of steroids should be started even if the biopsy cannot be performed for several days.

Less common causes of optic neuropathy include drug, tobacco, or alcohol toxicity; folic acid or vitamin B_{12} deficiency; and infections such as mumps, measles, and influenza. Pressure on the nerve from thyroid orbitopathy, tumors, or elevated intracranial pressure should be considered.

Meningioma is a tumor of the three layers of the membranes covering the brain. It is the most common central nervous system tumor and 90% are benign. Often causing no symptoms, they may be observed without treatment. Optic nerve sheath tumors are often followed without treatment unless there is visual loss (Fig. 118).

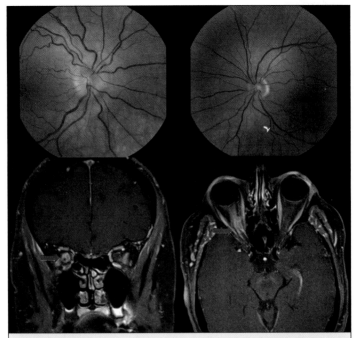

Fig. 118 CT scan of an optic nerve meningioma with secondary papilledema-like optic disk appearance. Unilateral congestion of the optic disk is due to obstruction of venous outflow from the eye and must be distinguished from papilledema, which is due to elevated intracranial pressure and causes bilateral blurring of disk margins. Courtesy of University of Iowa, Eyerounds.org.

Idiopathic intracranial hypertension (formally called pseudotumor cerebri) mainly affects young, overweight women of ages 20–40. Cerebrospinal fluid (CSF) pressure on the optic nerve may cause papilledema (Figs 443–447) followed by optic atrophy. Diagnosis is confirmed with CT scan, magnetic resonance imaging (MRI), and lumbar puncture. This spinal tap is positive with CSF pressure greater than 25 cmH$_2$O. Initial treatment includes weight loss, oral acetazolamide, and a low-sodium diet. If this conservative treatment is not successful, a shunt from a ventricle in the brain to the peritoneal cavity in the abdomen could lower the pressure. This is often the preferred treatment when headache is the main problem. Incision (fenestration) of the meninges surrounding the ipsilateral optic nerve may shunt CSF into the orbit and is often preferred when there is loss of vision due to pressure on the optic nerve.

The pupil

Both pupils are equally round and approximately 3–4 mm in diameter. Anisocoria refers to a difference in pupil size, and 4% of normal people may have a difference of as much as 1 mm. Miosis is a constricted pupil, and mydriasis is a dilated pupil. Pupil size is determined by a dilator muscle controlled by the sympathetic nerve and a constrictor muscle that has cholinergic innervation via CN III (Fig. 119).

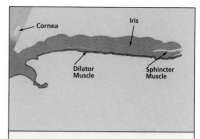

Fig. 119 Cross-section of anterior segment showing the iris-corneal junction, and the sphincter muscle (green) and dilator muscle (blue), which control pupil size. Courtesy of Pfizer Pharmaceuticals.

Sympathetic nerve

The iris dilator muscle and Müller's muscle that elevates the lid are both stimulated by the sympathetic nerve that begins in the hypothalamus (Fig. 120) and descends down the spinal column. At C8–T2 it synapses and then exits and passes over the apex of the lung. It ascends in the neck until it synapses, and follows the carotid artery into the skull and orbit. It dilates the pupil in response to the "fight or

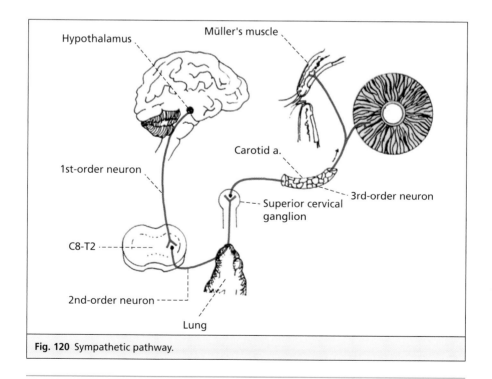

Fig. 120 Sympathetic pathway.

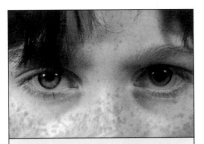

Fig. 121 Right Horner's syndrome. Associated neck pain on the same side is highly suggestive of a dissection of the wall of the carotid artery and should be referred immediately to the emergency room for vascular imaging. If caught early, anticoagulation may prevent a stroke (see Fig. 122).

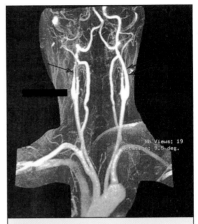

Fig. 122 Carotid artery dissection: magnetic resonance angiography (MRA) of right internal carotid (↑) shows decreased blood flow. Left internal carotid artery is normal (↑↑).

flight" stimulus. Damage to this nerve causes Horner's syndrome (Fig. 121): miosis, ptosis, and decreased sweating (anhidrosis).

Pupillary light reflex (Fig. 123)

Light shining on the retina stimulates the optic nerve and then the optic chiasm and optic tract. Here, it exits from the visual pathway to stimulate the Edinger–Westphal nucleus in the midbrain. The pupillary fibers leave the nucleus and travel with CN III until it synapses at the ciliary ganglion in the orbit. It innervates the iris sphincter muscle. Light shining in one eye causes that pupil and the pupil of the other eye to simultaneously constrict. The latter constriction is referred to as the consensual light reflex. Both pupils also constrict when the eye accommodates from distance to near. This normal state may be noted as PERRLA – pupils equally round and reactive to light and accommodation. An MRI of the brain, neck,

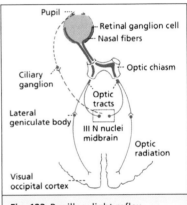

Fig. 123 Pupillary light reflex.

Causes of Horner's syndrome	
Neuron I	Spinal cord trauma, tumors, demyelinating disease, or syringomyelia
Neuron II	Apical lung tumors, goiter, neck injury, or surgery
Neuron III	Carotid dissection, migraine, cavernous sinus, or orbital disease

Causes of irregular pupils

Size of pupil

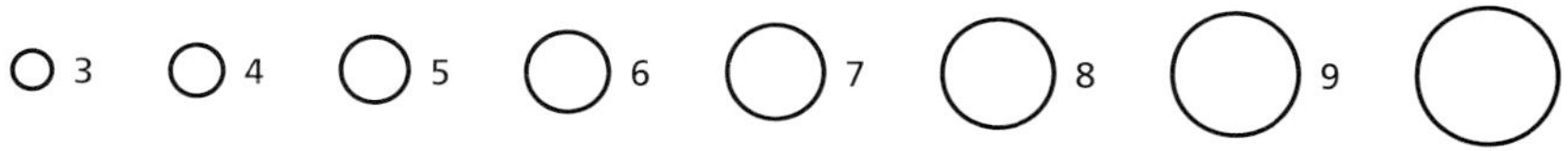

○ 3 ○ 4 ○ 5 ○ 6 ○ 7 ○ 8 ○ 9 ○ 10

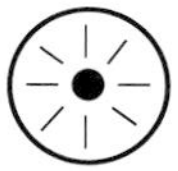

Miosis

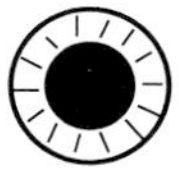

Mydriasis

↑ Cholinergic	↓ Sympathetic	Irritation to constrictor muscle	↓ Cholinergic	↑ Sympathetic	Damaged constrictor muscle
Pilocarpine drops used for glaucoma	Horner's syndrome	Iritis	Atropine	Phenylephrine	High eye pressure >40 mmHg
Morphine	Aldomet	Histamine release from inflammation	CN III paralysis	Epinephrine	Trauma (especially common with hyphemas)
	Reserpine		Adie's pupil	Anxiety	
			Antihistamines	Cocaine	
				Decongestants	

and upper chest should be considered when Horner's syndrome occurs. In children, rule out neuroblastoma when there are no other obvious causes such as birth trauma.

Adie's pupil (tonic pupil)

This is a dilated pupil with a reduced direct and consensual light reflex. It reacts slowly to accommodation, and eventually becomes smaller and stays smaller than the other eye, hence the name tonic pupil. It is due to a benign defect in the ciliary ganglion (Fig. 123). Resulting denervation hypersensitivity causes the tonic pupil to constrict intensely compared with the other eye in response to one drop of a weak cholinergic, such as pilocarpine 1/10%.

Visual field testing

The field of vision of each eye extends to 170° in the horizontal and 130° in the vertical meridian. Routine testing of vision with a Snellen chart recorded as 20/20 only means that the central 5° corresponding to the fovea and 17° of the macula are normal.

1 Amsler grid. This hand-held black crosshatched card tests the central 20° of the visual field. Waviness of lines is called metamorphopsia, and is characteristic of a wrinkled retina, which is especially common in wet macular degeneration (Fig. 124 and see also Appendix 2).

2 A tangent screen is a sheet of black felt (Fig. 125). It measures the central 60° of the field. The patient is seated 1 or 2 m from the screen with one eye occluded. The examiner moves a small white ball centrally until the patient first sees it. Areas blind to this small object are tested with progressively larger objects.

3 Hemisphere perimeters (Fig. 126) test the entire 170° of horizontal field and 130° of vertical field. Automated perimeters are expensive, but save examiner's time and give a record of the field. They project increasingly intense stimuli at one location until it is first seen.

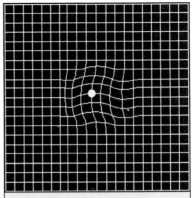

Fig. 124 Amsler grid. Distortion in wet macular degeneration.

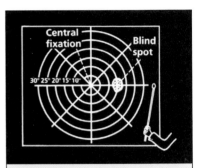

Fig. 125 Tangent screen tests the central 60°. It is useful when automated perimetry is too difficult to perform and to monitor enlargement of blind spot in papilledema.

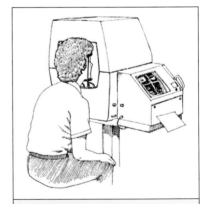

Fig. 126 An automated hemisphere perimeter tests central and peripheral fields.

4 Confrontation testing is a less accurate screen used when instruments aren't available. The patient is seated opposite the examiner. The patient closes his or her right eye, and each fixates on the other's open eye. The examiner moves an object in from the periphery and it should be seen simultaneously by both individuals. This technique compares the patient's and examiner's visual fields.

Scotomas due to ocular and optic nerve disease

A scotoma is loss of part of the visual field. Relative scotomas are areas of visual field blind to small objects, but able to perceive larger stimuli. Absolute scotomas are totally blind areas. Scintillating scotomas include sparkling lights (photopsias).

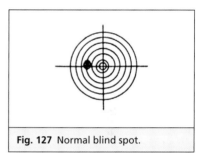

Fig. 127 Normal blind spot.

The normal blind spot is an absolute scotoma located 15° temporal to central fixation, which corresponds to the normal absence of rods and cones on the optic disk. It is plotted first (Fig. 127). If the blind spot cannot be located, the validity of the test should be considered.

Central scotomas (Fig. 128) occur in macular degeneration. Central and paracentral scotomas (Fig. 129) are most characteristic of optic nerve disorders.

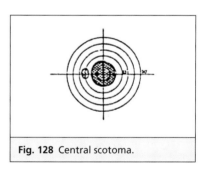

Fig. 128 Central scotoma.

Unilateral altitudinal scotomas are defects above or below the horizontal meridian and are most often caused by an occlusion of a superior or inferior retinal artery or vein and retinal detachment (Fig. 130).

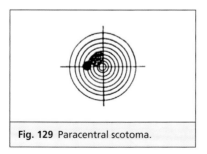

Fig. 129 Paracentral scotoma.

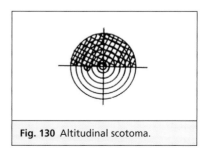

Fig. 130 Altitudinal scotoma.

Scotomas due to brain lesions

Field defects help to localize the site of brain lesions. Light focused on the temporal retina passes through the optic nerve and stimulates the occipital cortex on the same side, whereas fibers carrying impulses from the nasal retina cross over in the optic chiasm and stimulate the brain on the opposite side (see Fig. 131 and inner back cover). Therefore, defects at or posterior to the chiasm cause loss of vision in both eyes and respect the vertical meridian. If the defects are equal and on the same side, they are called homonymous (see table, notes 1, 4, and 5). If they are unequal on the same side, they are termed incongruous (note 3). If they are on opposite sides in each eye, they are referred to as bitemporal or binasal (note 2).

1	◗ ◖	The right homonymous hemianopsia is due to a lesion of the left occipital cortex.
2	◗ ◖	In the optic chiasm the nasal axons from each eye cross over (Fig. 131). Pituitary tumors (Fig. 132) press on these fibers and cause a bitemporal hemianopsia. Since the pituitary is also below the optic chiasm, the inferior-nasal fibers are more often affected. Bilateral superior-temporal defects are, therefore, most common.
3	◗ ◖	Optic tract lesions cause incongruous hemianopsia; that is, unequal in each eye.
4	◔ ◔	Optic radiation defects are often partial because the fibers are so widespread. A parietal lobe tumor that damages the superior half of the left radiation causes a right homonymous inferior quadrantopsia.
5	◗ ◖	Occipital cortex lesions usually cause a partial homonymous hemianopsia that is often vascular in origin, but tumors, trauma, and abscesses are also common (Figs 76 and 133)

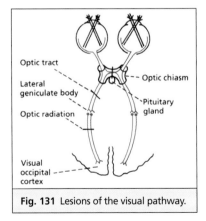

Fig. 131 Lesions of the visual pathway.

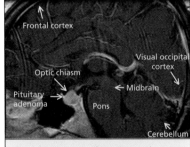

Fig. 132 CT scan of pituitary adenoma pressing on the optic chiasm which lies anterior and superior to it. Courtesy of Sandip Basak, MD.

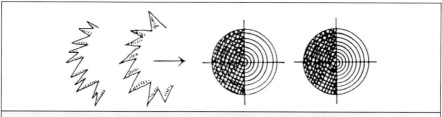

Fig. 133 Light flashes called scintillating scotomas are common in migraine. In this case, it progressed to a left homonymous hemianopsia.

Color vision

Color vision depends on the ability to see three primary colors: red, green, and blue. Partial defects are inherited in 7% of males and 0.5% of females and are detected using Ishihara or American optical pseudo-isochromatic plates. Loss of color vision could limit one's ability to become an electrician or airline pilot, or follow any profession requiring color discrimination. Acquired color defects may be due to retinal or optic nerve disease, the most common of which is optic neuritis. In acquired cases, test each eye separately and look for differences.

Circulatory disturbances affecting vision

The blood supply to the brain originates from the two carotid arteries in the antero-lateral neck and the two vertebral arteries passing through the cervical vertebrae (refer to Fig. 76). The circle of Willis interconnects these four arteries, helping distribute blood to all areas of the brain if one artery is obstructed. Transient loss of vision in persons younger than age 50 is often due to a migrainous spasm of a cerebral artery. This may be associated with brief flashes of light resembling zigzag lines (scintillations; Fig. 133) preceding a headache. It may progress to a homonymous hemianopsia lasting for 15–20 minutes. If neurologic symptoms persist, the patient should go to the emergency room.

In older persons, the transient blurring is more often due to arteriosclerosis and is referred to as a transient ischemic attack

(TIA), also called a "ministroke." The attack is caused by cholesterol, fibrin, or calcific emboli being liberated from plaques, most often in the carotid artery. Symptoms occur as these emboli pass through the eye or visual cortex of the brain and usually last less than a half hour, although the duration could be up to 24 hours. If it lasts longer, it could turn into a permanent obstruction called a stroke.

Five percent of TIAs go on to develop a stroke (cerebrovascular accident, CVA) within a month. So even if the symptoms have already cleared by the time the patient reaches your office, they should be cautioned about the risks of a permanent stroke and advised to see their primary care physician within a short time. If the TIA is still occurring after your examination, they should be sent directly to the emergency room since it could progress to a stroke. Eighty seven percent of strokes are ischemic due to emboli or thrombosis and 13% are hemorrhagic. The latter have a higher risk of fatality. In the emergency room the patient can be thoroughly evaluated to see if they meet the stringent guidelines to receive intravenous tissue plasminogen activator (tPA). There is a 3–4.5-hour therapeutic window from the onset of ischemic symptoms to administer this thrombolytic clot busting drug which could increase the chance of recovery from a stroke by 30–50% (Fig. 134). A CT scan is usually performed first in the emergency room to be sure it is ischemic and not hemorrhagic. Only then can tPA be safely administered.

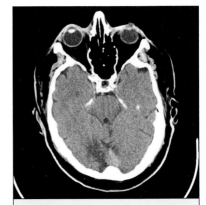

Fig. 134 MRI of right occipital infarct. Courtesy of Rand Kirkland, MD.

Tests for decreased circulation

Non-invasive duplex ultrasonography could show carotid stenosis and decreased blood flow. If positive, a CT angiogram may be ordered. Invasive arterial catheter angiography is infrequently used because there is a 1% chance of procedure-related stroke (Fig. 135), but it is still the gold standard. Carotid endarterectomy may be performed in symptomatic (high-risk) patients with 50% narrowing or in asymptomatic patients with 70% stenosis (see Appendix 1, Figs 545–547).

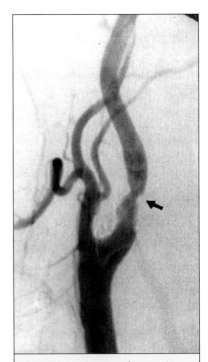

Fig. 135 Arteriogram of internal carotid artery narrowing.

	Carotid circulation	Posterior cerebral circulation
Cause	Cardiac abnormalities or carotid atheromas cause emboli to the retina and brain	Neck disorders affecting vertebral artery or emboli from atheroma
Symptoms	Unilateral curtain lasting a few minutes (amaurosis fugax): rarely headache, confusion, contralateral hemiparesis	Hemianopsia in both eyes: usually history of headache, dizziness, diplopia, drop attacks, or ringing in ears
Tests	An audible bruit over carotid artery in neck, duplex ultrasound, CT arteriogram, and cardiac evaluation	CT scan and MRI of brain (Fig. 134) with cardiac evaluation
Rx	Immediate thrombolysis (tPA), anticoagulants, endarterectomy, or stent	Immediate thrombolysis (tPA), anticoagulants, or stent

The right and left cavernous sinuses in the brain drain the superior and inferior ophthalmic veins from the orbit and face. Passing through the sinuses are the internal carotid artery, CN III–VI, and the sympathetic nerve (Fig. 136).

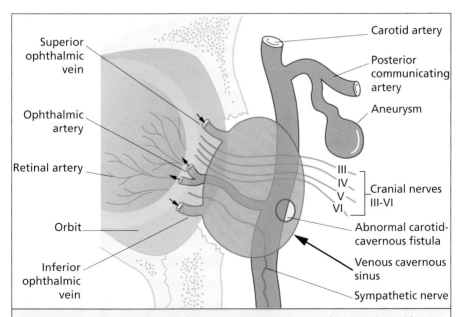

Fig. 136 Structures passing through the venous cavernous sinus are the internal carotid artery, CN III–VI, sympathetic nerve, superior and inferior ophthalmic veins, and retinal and ophthalmic arteries. Note the two abnormalities: (1) carotid-cavernous fistula and (2) the posterior communicating artery with its aneurysm pressing on CN III.

NEURO-OPHTHALMOLOGY   **49**

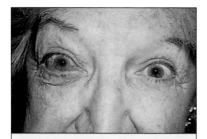

Fig. 137 Carotid-cavernous fistula.

Carotid-cavernous fistulas usually result from trauma to an aneurysm of the carotid artery in the cavernous sinus (Figs 137–139). It connects high-pressure arterial to low-pressure venous circulation causing a pulsating exophthalmos with a bruit over the eye, and tortuous – "corkscrew" – conjunctival vessels. Diagnosis is confirmed with carotid arteriography that shows an enlarged superior ophthalmic vein draining in a retrograde way towards the orbit, instead of towards the cavernous sinus.

It must be distinguished from a cavernous sinus thrombosis which causes a non-pulsatile exophthalmos. The latter is often due to infection carried to the sinus via the superior and inferior ophthalmic veins. An MRI is useful to show widening of the cavernous sinus. A carotid-cavernous fistula and a cavernous sinus thrombosis are two causes of exophthalmos that can mimic orbital cellulitis (Figs 211 and 212). What both conditions have in common with orbital cellulitis are conjunctival vascular engorgement and chemosis (Fig. 211); lids that are often swollen shut; and possible involvement of CN III–VI and the sympathetic nerve. Orbital cellulitis is usually unilateral; cavernous sinus thrombosis is commonly bilateral; and carotid-cavernous fistula is unilateral unless there are large connections between the right and left sinuses.

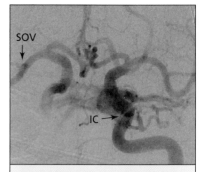

Fig. 138 Carotid-cavernous fistula causing bilateral CN VI palsies. Contrast injection into the femoral artery showing an enlarged superior ophthalmic vein (SOV) with retrograde flow and internal carotid artery (IC) within cavernous sinus.

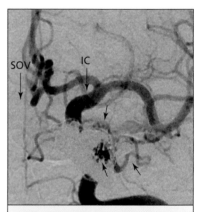

Fig. 139 Cerebral angiography through a femoral artery injection and passage of detachable platinum embolization coil through the superior ophthalmic vein located by a cutdown incision near the skinfold of the upper lid. Note the successful clouding of the obliterated cavernous sinus (↑) due to thrombosis and a narrowed superior ophthalmic vein (SOV) and uninterrupted blood flow through the distal internal carotid artery (IC) as it exits the sinus. Courtesy of Stavropoula I. Tjumakaris, MD, and Robert Rosenwasser, MD, Thomas Jefferson University Hospital.

Chapter 4
External structures

Begin with the four Ls: lymph nodes, lacrimal system, lids, and lashes.

Lymph nodes

Lymphatics from the lateral conjunctiva drain to the preauricular nodes just anterior to the ear. The nasal conjunctiva drains to the sub-mandibular nodes (Fig. 140). Enlarged or tender nodes help to distinguish infectious from allergic lid and conjunctival inflammations.

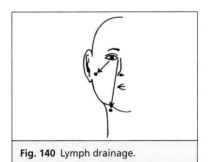

Fig. 140 Lymph drainage.

Lacrimal system

With each blink (once every 4 seconds) acting as a lacrimal pump, tears are moved nasally, where they enter the puncta and flow through the canaliculus, lacrimal sac, and the nasolacrimal duct (NLD) into the nose (Fig. 141). All eye drops are more effective and have less systemic side effects if patients press on the puncta and close the eyes for 60 seconds. This minimizes flow into the nose (Figs 142 and 143).

The tear film is made up of an outer oily component, a middle watery layer, and a

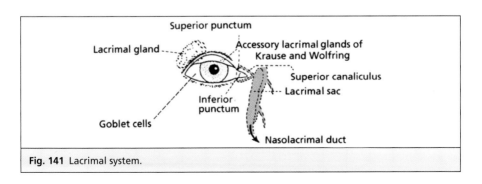

Fig. 141 Lacrimal system.

deep mucous layer (Fig. 144). A decrease in the oily, mucous, or watery tear could cause symptoms such as dryness, stinging, grittiness, sore eyes, blurry vision, and tearing from irritations. Dry eye disease (DED) is reported to affect 5% of the general population, 9% of menopausal women, and 34% of the elderly. With most external eye infections, the tear film is highly infectious. In AIDS, only bloody tears are so far considered infectious. In any case, wash your hands between patient examinations.

The oily layer is secreted by the meibomian glands in the lid and prevents dessication and lubricates the eyelids as they pass over the globe. Dysfunction of these glands occurs in almost half of Americans and often manifests with a toothpaste-like discharge (Figs 145 and 146) with occasional infection, referred to as posterior blepharitis. It is the most common reason for DED.

Watery tears provide anti-infective defenses, wash away debris, and smooth surface irregularities. Seventy percent is tonically secreted by the accessory lacrimal glands of Krause and Wolfring in the conjunctiva (Fig. 141). The lacrimal glands' contribution to watery tears is mostly a reflex response to emotion and ocular irritations. The corneal reflex arc has the trigeminal nerve (CN V) as its afferent pathway and the facial nerve as the efferent branch. Damage to the sensory CN V nerves causes dryness due to ocular surface changes and results from LASIK and PRK surgery, diabetic neurotrophic keratitis, and herpes simplex or zoster keratitis. Damage to the efferent CN VII, as in Bell's palsy, causes dessication due to incomplete blink reflex and inability to close the eye completely, especially at night. Corneal sensitivity (CN V) may be tested by touching a sterile cotton tip applicator to each eye and comparing blink reflexes. A wide variety of medications reduce watery tear production. They include diuretics and beta-blockers used to treat blood pressure, tranquilizers, antidepressants, antihistamines, anti-Parkinson disease drugs, bladder anti-spasmotics, and gastroprotective and gastric motility agents. A decrease in the

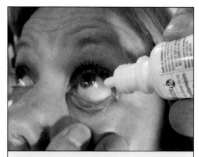

Fig. 142 Patients instill one drop by holding bottle like a pencil with one hand while the other hand pulls lower lid down as they look up. It is even easier if patient lies down to stabilize the head, but some prefer to look in a mirror.

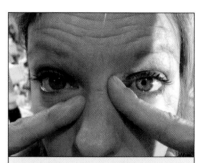

Fig. 143 After instilling drop, have patient push on upper and lower punctum for 60 seconds. This minimizes systemic side effects from drug entering nose and maximizes eye contact. Ask patient to show you their technique. The picture demonstrates the correct technique on the left side.

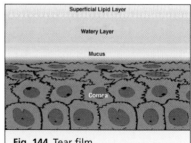

Fig. 144 Tear film.

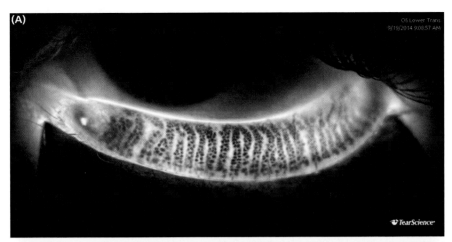

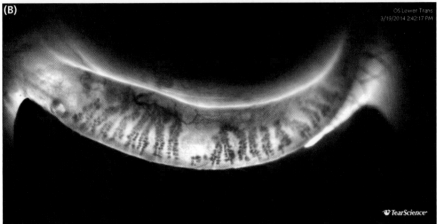

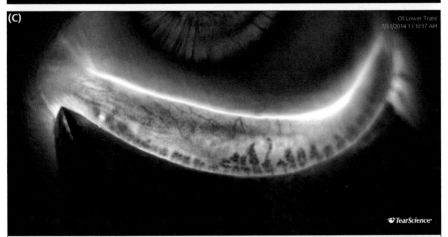

Fig. 145 Meibomian gland dysfunction demonstrated with transillumination of lid margin showing meibomian glands: (A) normal; (B) localized dropout; (C) severe dropout. Courtesy of LipiView II with DMI, TearScience.

watery mucous component could be due to aging or inflammation associated with systemic autoimmune diseases such as Sjögren's disease (dry eye, dry mouth, and arthritis). The resulting inflammatory ocular surface epithelial disease is called keratoconjunctivitis sicca. Fifty percent of Sjögren's patients have rheumatoid arthritis or lupus, both of which may also cause dry eye independent of Sjögren's. All three of these autoimmune diseases are often treated with hydroxychloroquinine.

Mucous is secreted by goblet cells and account for 5–20% of the conjunctival cells. The mucous traps exfoliated cells, bacteria, and other foreign bodies and washes them into the nose. Goblet cells decrease after menopause; or from any condition that damages the conjunctiva, such as Stevens–Johnson syndrome (Fig. 10), ocular pemphigoid (Fig. 282), trachoma (Fig. 287), alkalai burns (Figs 236 and 237), or vitamin A deficiency (Fig. 147). The latter could cause dysfunction of the conjunctival epithelial cells (Fig. 147) reducing both tears and mucous. Vitamin A deficiency could be due to poor diet or malabsorbtion which is surging due to the popularity of gastric bypass surgery used to treat obesity. Loss of vision from vitamin A deficiency may result from dessication of the cornea due to dryness or from decreased function of the rod receptors in the retina, which requires this vitamin to produce the visual pigment rhodopsin. Paradoxically, excess vitamin A is toxic and can cause elevated intracranial pressure with loss of vision (Fig. 447).

The diagnosis of DED may be confirmed by seeing punctate fluorescein staining of the corneal epithelial cells (Fig. 231) when illuminated by cobalt blue light. The integrity of the tear film layer is estimated by testing tear breakup time (TBUT) (Fig. 148). The Schirmer test measures tears on the surface of the eye. A drop of anesthetic is instilled and a strip of folded filter paper is placed on the surface of the conjunctiva (Fig. 149). Less than 10 mm of moist paper in 5 minutes is presumptive of a dry eye. Patients with dry eye have an abnormal Schirmer test 21% of

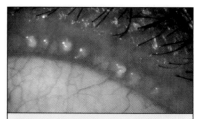

Fig. 146 There are 22 meibomian glands in both the upper and lower lid that normally secrete a clear, oily, meibum. In this case, the glands are dysfunctional with a white, pasty discharge. Courtesy of Michael Lemp, MD.

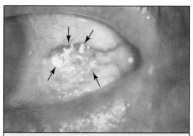

Fig. 147 A white Bitot's spot (↑) is due to conjunctival keratinization from vitamin A deficiency. These lesions appear in the perilimbal area. *Source*: Ahad MA et al., *Eye (Lond.)*, 2003, Vol. 17(5), pp. 671–673. Reprinted with permission of Macmillan Publishers.

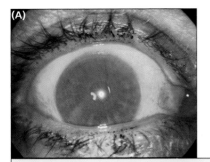

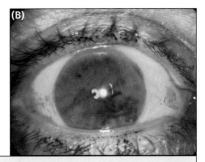

Fig. 148 Tear breakup time (TBUT). (A) Fluorescein placed on a normal cornea and observed with cobalt blue light has a uniform appearance. (B) With the lids held open, the pattern may abnormally break up before 10 seconds. Courtesy of Elliot Davidoff, MD.

the time, corneal staining with fluorescein 50% of the time, conjunctival staining with lissamine green, and an abnormal TBUT in 60% of cases. Lissamine green stain specifically stains devitalized conjunctival epithelium (Fig. 150).

Dry eye is treated in the daytime with artificial tears and at night with ointments. There are many on the market and vary mostly by their viscosity, cost, and whether they have preservatives. The patient decides which one is best. Unfortunately, symptomatic relief lasts only 10–15 minutes, often leading to excessive use. If annoying symptoms persist, the puncta may be closed with absorbable or permanent punctal plugs (Fig. 151), resulting in more

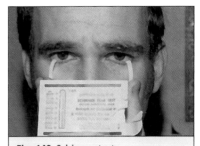

Fig. 149 Schirmer test.

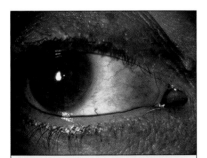

Fig. 150 Lissamine green stain of devitalized conjunctival epithelial cells. The density of stain increases in dry eye and is usually in the interpalpebral area. Courtesy of Eric Donnenfeld, MD, NYU Medical Center.

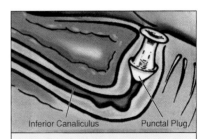

Inferior Canaliculus   Punctal Plug

Fig. 151 Punctal plug. Problems include 40% loss of plugs, 9% epiphora, and 10% ocular irritation, especially from the inability to flush toxic and inflammatory chemicals from the surface of the eye. Courtesy of Eagle Vision.

than 50% improvement. Room humidifiers may be tried and oral flaxseed oil increases meibomian gland secretions. Since computer use and reading suppress blinking and aggravate DED, intentional blinking should be encouraged. Restasis (cyclosporine ophthalmic emulsion) 0.05% eye drops used twice a day may increase tear production by suppressing lymphocyte T-cell-induced inflammation. Low-dose steroid eye drops, such as fluorometholone (FML, 0.19%) are infrequently added. DED may cause corneal changes, resulting in fluctuating vision. It is critical to document its presence before corneal refractive or cataract surgery, which could aggravate the condition and thus cause patient disgruntlement.

Tearing (epiphora)

Tearing is a very common complaint and is often minor enough so as not to require the workup and treatment discussed below.

There are two causes of tearing (epiphora):

1 increased tear production due to emotion and eye irritation; paradoxically, dry eye stimulates reflex tearing;
2 tears that are produced normally but which cannot flow properly into the nose.

Tearing due to failure of drainage system

Once increased tear production is ruled out as the cause of tearing, an evaluation is made of the patency of the ducts leading into the nose. An obstruction is presumed if fluorescein dye placed on the conjunctiva (Fig. 152) disappears slowly and asymmetrically from one eye, or runs over the lid onto the cheek.

Failure of the tear to reach the puncta

This could be due to horizontal laxity of the lower lid which decreases the pumping action of the blink reflex, or an everted puncta, as occurs in an ectropion (Fig. 165), in which case the tear lake is not in contact with the

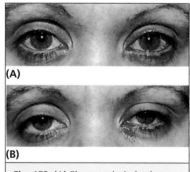

(A)

(B)

Fig. 152 (A) Fluorescein in both eyes. (B) Obstruction prevents exit of dye in left eye.

punctal orifice. Either can often be corrected by surgically tightening the lower lid with a full-thickness wedge resection.

Obstruction at the puncta or canaliculus

The puncta may become narrowed due to aging, topical drugs, trauma, and infections, especially from blepharitis.

The puncta and canaliculi can be dilated with progressively wider-diameter punctal probes (Fig. 153). If the lumen is still inadequate, a snip incision can widen the puncta. If still unsuccessful, a self-retaining bicanalicular stent (Fig. 154) can be inserted in the office with topical anesthetic and left in place for 3 months. If epiphora is primarily due to canalicular failure, a Pyrex glass tube may be permanently inserted, creating a fistula from the conjunctiva to the nasal cavity. Traumatic laceration of the canaliculus can be repaired using a pigtail probe (Fig. 155). The probe is passed through the upper puncta toward the laceration. A silicone tube is threaded onto it and is withdrawn. The probe is then passed through the lower puncta and the other end of the silicone tube is threaded onto it and is withdrawn, forming a continuous lumen to heal over the tube.

Rarely, the canaliculus can be obstructed due to an *Actinomyces israelii* infection. In this case, incise the canaliculus and remove sand-like concretions. This bacterium is sensitive to penicillin and sulfa drugs.

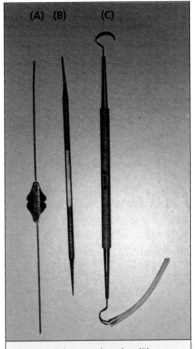

Fig. 153 (A) Punctal probe. (B) Punctum dilator. (C) Pigtail probe.

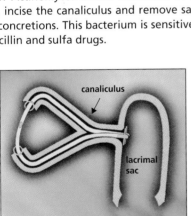

Fig. 154 Bicanalicular stent for puncta stenosis or canalicular constriction. Courtesy of FCI Ophthalmics.

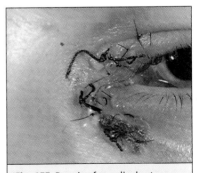

Fig. 155 Repair of canalicular tear.

Tearing due to NLD obstructions

In adults, obstructions result from chronic nasal inflammation. In infants, the distal opening of this duct in the nose – called the valve of Hasner – fails to open at birth. Although 90% spontaneously open by 1 year of age, repeated infections may mandate treatment at 6–12 months. In these infants, the puncta may be irrigated and/or probed to the nose (Figs 156 and 157). The same technique can be used in adults. If it is still narrowed, a balloon catheter may be used to widen the passage (Fig. 158), and/or a silicone stent may be inserted through the puncta, canaliculus, and the NLD into the nose and left in place for 2–4 months.

If it still remains closed, a new surgical opening in the nasal bone is created and the mucosa of the lacrimal sac is sutured to the nasal mucosa (dacryocystorhinostomy). Besides tearing, an additional motivation for performing the latter surgical procedure is recurring infections of the lacrimal sac (dacryocystitis; Fig. 159), caused by stagnant tear flow.

Signs of dacryocystitis are swelling and tenderness over the lacrimal sac with pus exuding from the puncta when pressure is applied to the sac. Rx: massage the sac, nasal decongestant, local (see table) and systemic antibiotics, then a dacryocystorhinostomy to open the NLD.

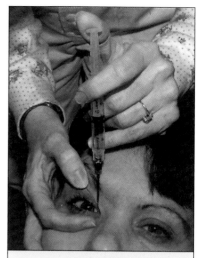

Fig. 156 Irrigation of NLD.

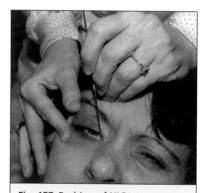

Fig. 157 Probing of NLD.

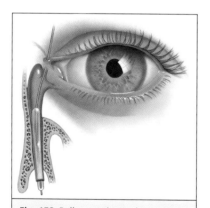

Fig. 158 Balloon catheter dacryoplasty: inflate the balloon with sterile saline. Courtesy Quest Medical, Inc.

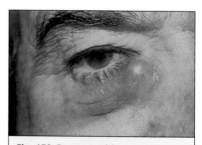

Fig. 159 Dacryocystitis.

Common topical anti-infectives

Trade name	Generic name
Antibiotic	
Bleph 10%	Sulfacetamide 10%
Ciloxan solution or ointment	Ciprofloxin 0.3%
Ilotycin 0.5% ointment	Erythromycin ointment 0.5%
Gentac solution or ointment	Gentamycin 0.3%
Neosporin solution	Neomycin, polymixin B, gramicidin
Neosporin ointment	Neomycin, polymyxin, bacitracin
Ocuflox solution	Ofloxacin 0.3%
Polytrim solution	Polymixin B, trimethoprim sulfate
Polysporin ointment	Polymixin B, bacitracin
Tobrex solution or ointment	Tobramycin 0.3%
Antibiotic/steroid combination	
Blephamide suspension or ointment	Sulfacetamide 10%, prednisolone 0.2%
Cortisporin suspension	Neomycin, polymixin B, hydrocortisone
Maxitrol solution or Oint	Neomycin, polymixin B, dexamethasone
Poly-Pred suspension or ointment	Prednisolone, neomycin, polymixin B
Tobradex solution or ointment	Tobramycin 0.3%, dexamethasone 0.1%
Vasocidin solution or ointment	Sulfacetamide 10%, prednisolone 0.5%

Lids

Lid swelling is commonly due to allergy, in which case the edema clears with a telltale shriveling of the skin between episodes (Fig. 160). Dependent edema, caused by body fluid retention, affects the lids on awakening and the ankles later in the day. Test for the latter by indenting the pretibial area of the lower leg seeing if there is a prolonged pitting. Traumatic causes are also common. Less frequently, it is due to hypothyroidism (myxedema) and orbital venous congestion due to orbital masses or cavernous sinus thrombosis or fistulas.

Dermatochalasis is loose skin (Fig. 161) due to aging, and is aggravated by recurrent bouts of lid edema due to stretching of the skin. There may be palpable orbital fat that has herniated

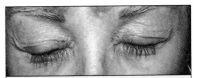

Fig. 160 Shriveled skin following allergy.

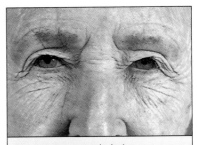

Fig. 161 Dermatochalasis.

through the orbital septum (Figs 162 and 163). A surgical blepharoplasty is performed for cosmetic reasons or if the resulting drooping of the lid (ptosis) obstructs vision.

Lid-margin lacerations must be carefully approximated to prevent notching. Pass a 4-0 silk suture through both edges of the tough tarsal plate using the grey line for accurate alignment (Fig. 164).

An ectropion (Fig. 165) is an outturned lid. It is often caused by senile relaxing of the lid. This is aggravated in patients who chronically dab their tears or apply eye drops, since both cause downward tugging and weakening of lid tissue. Less common causes are CN VII paralysis or traction of scarred skin on the lower lid. Correct with surgery.

An entropion (Fig. 166) is an inturned lid margin. It may be due to contraction of scarred conjunctiva (Fig. 10), senile lid laxity, or spasm of the orbicularis oculi muscle. It is corrected with surgery. The palpebral fissure is the space between the upper and lower lid (Fig. 167). Differences in the size of the

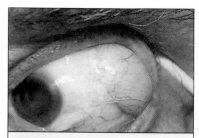

Fig. 162 Orbital fat under conjunctiva.

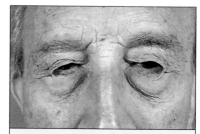

Fig. 163 Prolapsed fat through septum is palpable beneath lower lid.

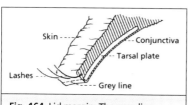

Fig. 164 Lid margin. The grey line delineates the mucocutaneous junction.

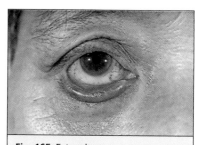

Fig. 165 Ectropion.

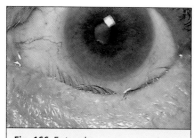

Fig. 166 Entropion.

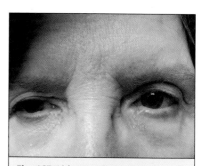

Fig. 167 Lid retraction in Grave's disease causing the left eye to appear larger.

palpebral fissures occur with ptosis (droopy lid), lid retraction in thyroid disease, exophthalmos (protruding eye), or enophthalmos (sunken eye). If the fissure is larger on one side, it gives the appearance of one eye looking larger than the other, but is almost never due to disparity in the size of of the globe. Rare exception is an enlarged globe in congenital glaucoma (Fig. 343) and a severely damaged shrunken globe (phthis bulbi).

Blepharoptosis (also called ptosis)

Ptosis refers to a drooping lid with narrowing of the palpebral fissure. It may be present at birth, in which case it is usually due to underaction of the levator muscle. It is followed without surgery if it does not obstruct vision or is not cosmetically disfiguring.

Surgical correction of the ptosis depends on the amount of levator muscle function still present. With good levator muscle action, an advancement of the muscle on the tarsal plate is sufficient (Figs 168–171). Sometimes, one must also resect a piece of the muscle, which further tightens it. With little levator function, as in congenital ptosis, a frontalis slight operation is performed where the

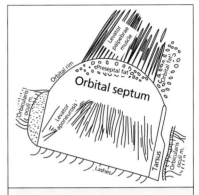

Fig. 168 The orbital septum, originating at the superior orbital rim, thickens to form the tarsal plate. The levator palpebral muscle originates in the orbital apex. Its aponeurosis then passes through and inserts onto the anterior tarsal plate. The orbicularis muscle that closes the lids overlies the levator muscle and its fibers must be split to expose the levator muscle.

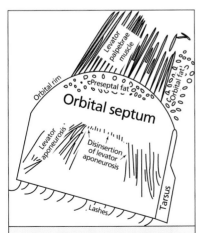

Fig. 169 Partial disinsertion of the levator palpebral aponeurosis from the tarsal plate.

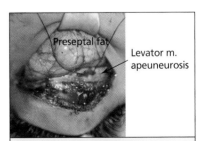

Fig. 170 Repair of ptosis by surgically advancing the levator palpebrae aponeurosis and suturing it to the inferior tarsus.

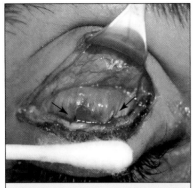

Fig. 171 Disinserted levator aponeurosis in Fig. 170 sutured to inferior tarsus. Courtesy of Joseph A. Mauriello, Jr., MD.

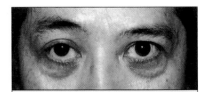

Fig. 172 Myasthenia gravis: no ptosis.

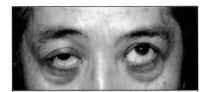

Fig. 173 Myasthenia gravis: ptosis after looking up for 5 minutes.

tarsal plate is connected to the frontalis muscle above the brow.

Periodically occurring ptosis by itself, or with diplopia, may be the first sign of myasthenia gravis. In this myoneural junction disorder, the ptosis may worsen when tired, or after a provocative test such as asking the patient to look up for several minutes (Figs 172 and 173).

Other neurologic causes of ptosis are CN III paralysis (Figs 92–94) and sympathetic nerve dysfunction (Figs 120 and 121).

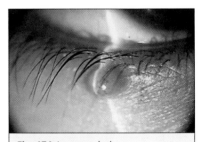

Fig. 174 Ingrown lash.

Lashes

Trichiasis (inturned lashes) causes corneal irritations, and may be the result of an entropion (inturned lid) (Figs 166 and 234), or trauma to the lid margin. Lashes can be epilated (pulled out), or the lash follicles can be destroyed with electrolysis or cryosurgery.

Lashes sometimes grow under the skin (Fig. 174) and may be removed after injection of local anesthetic.

Lice (pediculosis capitis) on the scalp, hair, and lashes cause blepharitis and conjunctivitis (Fig. 175). There are 6 million cases a year in the USA, mainly in children aged 3–12. Rx:

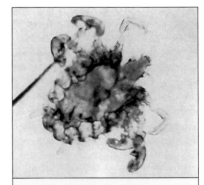

Fig. 175 Crab louse.

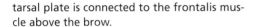

if over-the-counter permethrin shampoo is ineffective, use the more toxic lindane 1% by prescription.

Madarosis refers to loss of eyelashes and/ or eyebrows. It may be due to skin disease, trauma, blepharitis, and epilation due to psychiatric reasons (trichotillomania).

Verrucas (warts) (Fig. 176), caused by the papilloma virus, and molluscum contagiosum (Figs 177 and 178), caused by the pox virus, are both common skin lesions. When close to the eye, both should be considered as a cause for chronic conjunctivitis not responsive to usual treatment. They are often multifocal and easily spread to surrounding tissues (see Fig. 281, p. 91, for conjunctival verruca). Excision is usually performed for cosmetic reasons and to prevent proliferation. Cases of molluscum are usually treated with curettage of the central umbilicated dimple. The verruca is excised with cauterization of the base.

Seborrheic keratosis (Fig. 179), which is common with aging, is a benign, brown, rough-surfaced growth appearing stuck on, like clay thrown against a wall. It is excised for cosmetic reasons.

Epidermoid inclusion cysts (Fig. 180) are intracutaneous benign, smooth, glistening, white balls filled with cheesy substance and are also excised for cosmetic reasons.

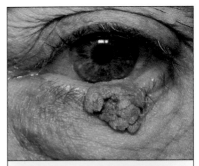

Fig. 176 Verruca vulgaris (wart) with its typical cauliflower-like appearance. Courtesy of Michael Stanley, Medical College of Georgia.

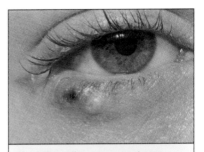

Fig. 177 Molluscum contagiosum are small, firm, rounded umbilicated papules with caseous material in the center. They may be single or multiple. Courtesy of Malcolm Luxemberg, MD, and *Arch. Ophthalmol.*, Sept. 1986, Vol. 104, p. 1390. Copyright 1986, American Medical Association. All rights reserved.

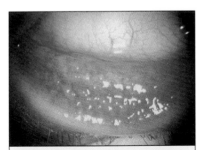

Fig. 178 Follicular conjunctivitis due to viral molluscum contagiosum. Courtesy of Malcolm Luxemberg, MD, and *Arch Ophthalmol.*, Sept. 1986, Vol. 104, p. 1390. Copyright 1986, American Medical Association. All rights reserved.

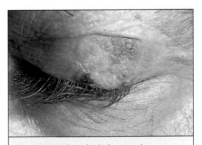

Fig. 179 Seborrheic keratosis.

Nevi (Fig. 181) are benign, non-pigmented or pigmented, well-demarcated growths present from early childhood. Suspect malignancy if there is growth, irregular edges, inflammation, satellites, irregular pigment, ulceration, or bleeding.

Keratoacanthoma (Fig. 182) is a benign growth that resolves spontaneously. Rolled edges with an umbilicated center filled with keratin make it difficult to distinguish from carcinoma, so a biopsy is sometimes indicated.

Infantile hemangiomas (Fig. 183) are the most common, benign tumors of the lid and orbit in children. They appear shortly after birth, affecting 1–3% of infants, and often regress by 2–3 years of age. Treatment is necessary if it causes the lid to block vision or if it causes strabismus or compression of the globe. Systemic or intralesional corticosteroids are often the preferred regimen, but removal using a laser or scalpel are possible. Systemic or topical beta-blockers may be tried.

The lids, face, and scalp are the most common locations for basal cell carcinoma, and, less often, squamous cell carcinoma, of the skin (Fig. 184). The lids alone account for 5–10% of all skin cancers. They are strongly related to the cumulative exposure to the sun's ultraviolet rays. Therefore, sunbathing should be discouraged at all ages, especially in fair-skinned people. Basal and squamous cell carcinomas are the most common malignancies in humans, occurring in 1 in 5 Americans. All chronic, hard, nodular, umbiliated, ulcerated, vascularized lesions demand a biopsy.

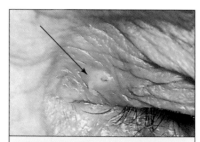
Fig. 180 Epidermoid inclusion cyst.

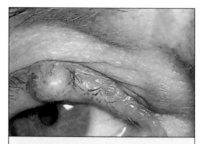
Fig. 181 Nevus.

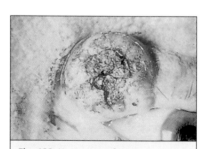
Fig. 182 Keratoacanthoma.

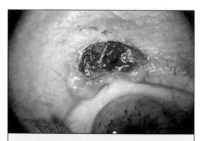
Fig. 184 Carcinoma of the lid is usually basal cell, but squamous cell looks similar and is also common.

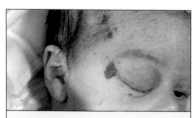
Fig. 183 Infantile hemangioma.

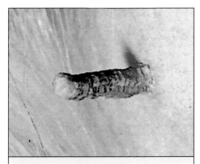

Fig. 185 Cutaneous horn.

Cutaneous horns (Fig. 185) are keratinized overgrowths of seborrheic keratosis, verruca, or squamous or basal cell carcinoma; therefore, a biopsy of the base is indicated.

Phakomatoses

Congenital syndromes that include lesions of the brain, skin, and eye are called phakomatoses. The early onset of skin lesions in these infants and young children provide a red flag to alert one to other problems.

1 Tuberous sclerosis is a condition appearing in the first 3 years of life. Patients may manifest seizures, mental deficiency, and sebaceous adenoma. Seventy five percent die before age 20 (Figs 186 and 187).
2 Sturge–Weber syndrome includes facial port wine capillary malformations (Fig. 188) and mental retardation in half of the patients. They should be monitored for early onset glaucoma or choroidal and central nervous system (CNS) hemangiomas.
3 Neurofibromatosis is a condition that is inherited in an autosomal dominant pattern with incomplete penetrance. Tumors could affect the optic nerve, iris, retina, and skin of the lid (Fig. 189). Lisch nodules in the iris are present in 94% of patients (Fig. 190). Brown macular skin lesions occur early on and eventually in 99% in patients.

Leprosy is a chronic disease caused by acid-fast *Mycobacterium leprae*. It is probably transmitted by the respiratory route and usually involves prolonged exposure in childhood (Figs 191 and 192).

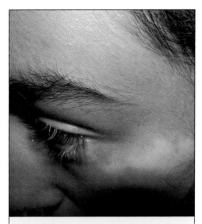

Fig. 186 Ash-leaf spots on the skin are multiple, depigmented macules with irregular borders. They are usually the first sign of tuberous sclerosis and appear in up to 90% of patients.

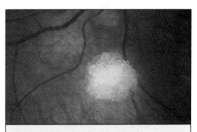

Fig. 187 Retinal astrocytoma in tuberous sclerosis. Areas of calcification give mulberry appearance. Courtesy of Dana Gabel, Barnes Retinal Institute, St. Louis, MO.

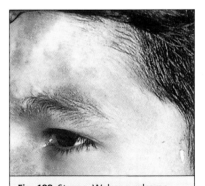

Fig. 188 Sturge–Weber syndrome.

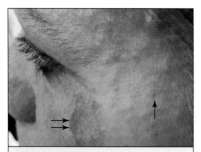

Fig. 189 Neurofibromatosis (von Recklinghausen disease) is characterized by neurofibromas of the skin (↑) and nervous system, and café-au-lait spots (↓↓), which are irregularly shaped brown macules. There are usually multiple (five or more) increasing in size from 0.5 to 1.5 cm in adults.

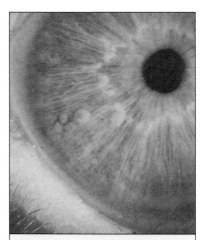

Fig. 190 Lisch nodues on the iris of a patient with neurofibromatosis. Courtesy of S.J. Charles, FRCS, and *Arch. Ophthalmol.*, Nov. 1989, Vol. 107, p. 1572. Copyright 1989, American Medical Association. All rights reserved.

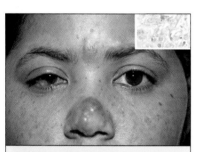

Fig. 191 Twenty two year-old from Cape Verde Islands with lepromatous leprosy. There are macular and erythematous nodular lesions on face, trunk, and extremities. Fite's stain/acid-fast bacilli in skin biopsy confirms the diagnosis.

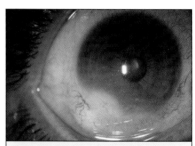

Fig. 192 Leprosy causing a solid nodule on the ocular surface together with granulomatous iritis. Courtesy of Carly Seidman, BS, and *Arch. Ophthalmol.*, Dec. 2010, Vol. 128, p. 1522. Copyright 2010, American Medical Association. All rights reserved.

Anterior and posterior blepharitis

Blepharitis refers to inflammation or infection of the lid margin. It is extremely common and is reported to occur in up to 50% of adults. There is rarely a day that goes by that an eye doctor doesn't treat it or one of its sequelae, such as conjunctivitis, sties, chalazia, corneal ulcers, lid cellulitis, dry eye, or intolerance to contact lenses.

Infections of the cornea, conjunctiva, and lid margins can usually be treated with relatively inexpensive generic antibiotic eye drops and ointments (see table above, Common topical anti-infectives). A lot of thought has gone into giving brand medications short, easy-to-remember names without having to write all components and concentrations. Writing these brand names, and approving the generic form on the prescription, saves time and increases accuracy. Sometimes, the generic name, such as bacitracin or erythromycin ointment (see table, p. 59), is more convenient.

Anterior blepharitis manifests with crusting, redness, and ulcerative lesions around the lashes (Figs 193 and 194). Infections are usually due to staphylococcal bacteria. The seborrheic type, associated with dandruff of the scalp and eyebrows, responds to appropriate shampoos.

A less common type is caused by the *Demodex* mite (demodex blepharitis). This member of the spider family inhabits the lashes of almost all adults. Some people are more sensitive and get itching and conjunctivitis. It can be detected at the slit lamp by noting cylindrical cuffs around the base of the lashes (Fig. 196). There are commercial tea tree preparations available (Cliradex and Demodex®) to treat this infestation.

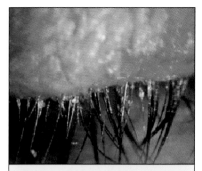

Fig. 193 Anterior blepharitis with crusting flakes on lashes. Courtesy of Michael Lemp, MD.

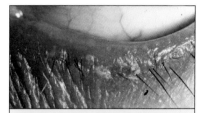

Fig. 194 Anterior blepharitis with crusting and ulcerative lesions around lashes. Courtesy of Michael Lemp, MD.

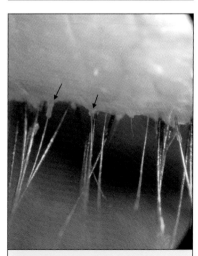

Fig. 196 Demodex blepharitis is identified by a telltale cylindrical cuff around the base of eyelash (↑). Compare with pediculosis capitus which is a different lid infestation in which the parasite and eggs (nits) are seen at slit lamp (Fig. 175). Courtesy of Eric Donnenfeld, MD, NYU Medical Center.

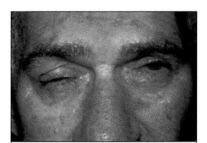

Fig. 195 Blepharoconjunctivitis in acne rosacea. This chronic condition is associated with engorged vessels and pustules on the nose, forehead, cheeks, and chin.

Posterior blepharitis (Figs 197–199) may involve all 22 meibomian glands on both the upper and lower lids. These glands often become dysfunctional, losing their ability to produce the meibum which contributes the oily portion of the tear film (Figs 145 and 146). It's been reported that up to 86% of dry eyes are due in part to this disorder. It is often associated with acne rosacea (Fig. 195). White heads on the meibomian orifices (Fig. 197) and foamy residue (Fig. 199) are abnormal clues.

Anterior and posterior blepharitis often occur together (Fig. 200). Both require good lid hygiene, including warm soaks and mechanical scrubs for which over-the-counter antibacterial cleaning solutions are available. Less expensive baby shampoo may be used. These conditions are often chronic and maintenance of preventive therapy between attacks should be encouraged.

For more resistant cases, commercially available lid-margin cleansing solutions containing up to 0.02% hypochlorous acid (Avenosa) are available by prescription. Antibiotic drops or ointment may be added (see table, p. 59, on Common topical anti-infectives). Nonsteroidal anti-inflammatory drugs (NSAIDs), such as ketorolac 0.5%, are sometimes needed. Steroids may be added with caution, since gritty, sore eyes with fluorescein staining of the cornea are common to both blepharitis and herpes keratitis. Oral generic antibiotics, such as doxycycline 100 mg BID, is used when symptoms include blurry vision, keratitis, lid cellulitis (Fig. 204), or corneal ulcers.

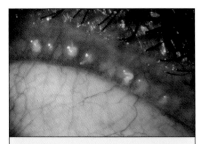

Fig. 197 Toothpaste-like meibum spontaneously exuding from glands make for an easy diagnosis. Courtesy of Eric Donnenfeld, MD, NYU Medical Center.

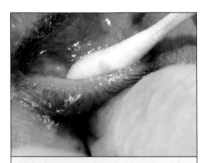

Fig. 198 Posterior blepharitis: dysfunctional meibomian glands may be diagnosed by massaging the lid and and revealing a toothpaste-like secretion. It is also therapeutic.

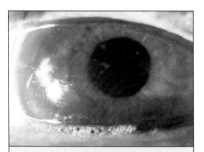

Fig. 199 Posterior blepharitis with foamy residue overlying the meibomian glands. Courtesy of Michael Lemp, MD.

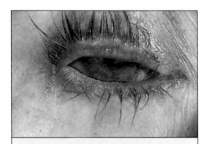

Fig. 200 Anterior and posterior blepharitis often occur together.

The lid margin may be massaged to reveal a diagnostic white paste, instead of the usual clear oil. The patient should be told that this sometimes uncomfortable procedure is also therapeutic (Fig. 198). Many get significant relief and return at regular intervals requesting massage.

Chalazia (Fig. 201) are cystic enlargements of the meibomian glands that occur due to clogging of an orifice. Retention of lipid and its breakdown by-products incite a granulomatous inflammatory reaction. They are usually painless, unless infected. As with blepharitis, treatment includes warm compresses and lid scrubs. Antibiotic/steroid drops (see table, p. 59), or even intralesional steroid injections, with or without antibiotic, are often considered. Oral generic doxycycline with incision and drainage are sometimes needed (Fig. 202).

Sties are infections of the glands of Zeis and Moll around the lashes (Fig. 203). These pimples are treated with hot soaks, local antibiotics, and incision. Systemic antibiotics are indicated if there is significant surrounding cellulitis.

Lid cellulitis is a diffuse infection often due to a sty, chalazion, bug bite, or cut. Lids are red and tender (Figs 204 and 210). There may be adenopathy and fever. Rx: topical and systemic antibiotics. Shriveled skin, as in Fig. 160, is an initial indication that lid cellulitis is responding to treatment. Be cautious. When severe, it can penetrate the orbital septum (see Figs 205, 211, and 212 in the next chapter), resulting in orbital cellulitis that could extend into the brain, causing meningitis and even death.

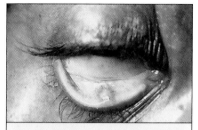

Fig. 201 Chalazia point internally.

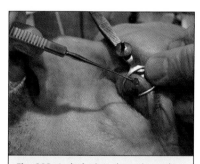

Fig. 202 A chalazion clamp is used to minimize bleeding during incision and curettage.

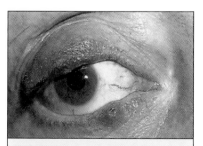

Fig. 203 Sties point externally.

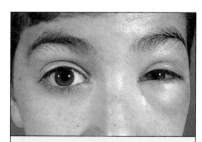

Fig. 204 Preseptal cellulitis – i.e., in front of orbital septum (Figs 168 and 205) – typically affects chidren and is usually secondary to lid infections. Orbital cellulitis most often originates from infections behind the orbital septum, most commonly in the sinuses.

Chapter 5
The orbit

The orbit is a cone-shaped vault (Figs 205 and 206). At its apex are three orifices through which pass the nerves, arteries, and veins supplying the eye.

Unlike the eye, in which most parts are amenable to direct visualization, evaluation of the orbit often requires the use of diagnostic tools such as CT scans and MRI. CT scans are usually the radiologic technique of choice to evaluate orbital diseases such as fracture, foreign bodies, thyroid disease (Figs 1–3) and sinusitis (Figs 207–209).

CT scanning has made amazing contributions to medical diagnosis, but it is a large

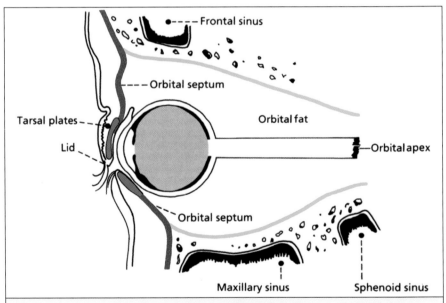

Fig. 205 Side view of orbit; periosteum (periorbital) of the orbit (green), the orbit septum (red), and tarsal plate (blue) are continuous connective tissue membranes. This fibrous membrane then goes on to cover the optic nerve as it exits the orbit and is continuous with the dura mater covering the brain.

Manual for Eye Examination and Diagnosis, Ninth edition. Mark Leitman.

70 © 2017 John Wiley & Sons, Inc. Published 2017 by John Wiley & Sons, Inc.

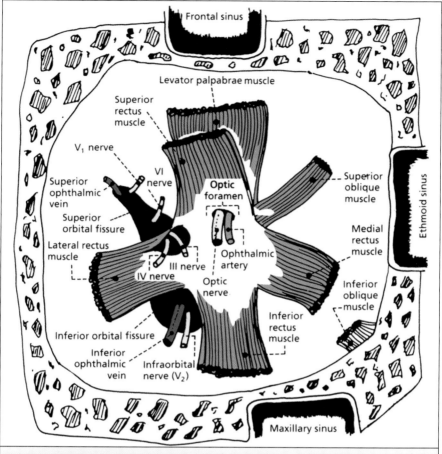

Fig. 206 Front view shows the apex of the orbit.

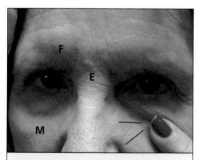

Fig. 207 One piece of evidence for sinusitis is to elicit tenderness by palpating over the frontal (F), ethmoid (E), or maxillary (M) sinus. In this case, the left maxillary sinus is involved.

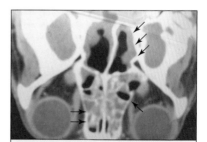

Fig. 208 CT showing three typical findings of ethmoiditis. A level flat surface of fluid accumulation (↑) and opacification of the air spaces (↑↑) are common in an acute process. Thickening of mucosal membrane is more typical of chronicity (↑↑↑).

contributor to the six-fold increase in diagnostic radiation in the last 30 years, because of overutilization. It is predicted that CT scans may be responsible for 1.5–2.0% of all future cancers in the USA and studies reveal that patients are not informed of this risk 90–95% of the time.

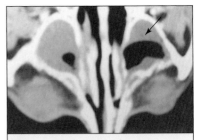

Fig. 209 CT scan of sphenoidal sinusitis with air-fluid level (↑).

Sinusitis

The orbit is surrounded on four sides by the periorbital paranasal sinuses; i.e., the maxillary, frontal, sphenoid, and ethmoid sinuses. Pain, described as deep, or behind the eye, is most often due to allergy or infection of these sinuses. Pressure applied to the skin overlying the inflamed frontal, maxillary, and ethmoidal sinuses may cause tenderness (Fig. 207). The sphenoid sinus is behind the globe and cannot be tested in this way.

Clues that may indicate disease of the orbit

1 Proptosis (exophthalmos): forward bulging of the eye.
2 Enophthalmos: sunken eye.
3 Swollen lids (sometimes totally shut); redness and engorgement of conjunctival vessels; clear fluid under conjunctiva (chemosis).
4 Loss of eye movement (ophthalmoplegia) due to involvement of CN III, IV, and VI or local damage to extraocular muscles.
5 Rare elevation of intraocular pressure due to venous congestion.

Preseptal cellulitis causes swollen lids which may be totally shut (Figs 204 and 210). This may progress to the rarer and more serious orbital cellulitis (Figs 211 and 212), in which case the globe may not move (ophthalmoplegia) and there is chemosis, fever, adenopathy, and exophthalmos. It is due to sinusitis 60% of the time, but also occurs with tooth, facial, or lid infections.

A tough connective tissue called the periorbita lines the inner surface of the orbit.

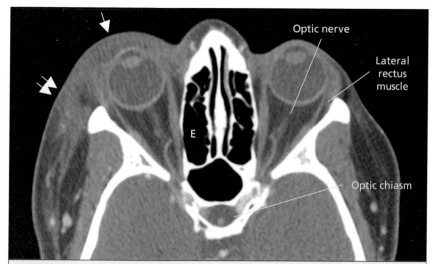

Fig. 210 CT scan showing preseptal lid swelling (↑) and periorbital cellulitis (↑↑). The retrobulbar areas of the orbit and the ethmoid (E) sinuses are normal. There are, as yet, normal eye movements and no proptosis. Mild, early cases could be followed up cautiously on an outpatient basis. Courtesy of Sandip Basak, MD.

At the orbital rim, it becomes the orbital septum which then thickens to become the tarsal plate of the lid (see Figs 168 and 205). This continuous fibrous membrane acts as a barrier protecting the orbit from lid and sinus infections and might be considered an "orbital firewall." Beware of the rare breakthrough. If orbital cellulitis occurs, it can easily spread to the cavernous sinus through the superior and inferior ophthalmic veins that drain the orbit and part of the face. This can cause thrombosis and death. Hospitalize the patient and treat with systemic antibiotics.

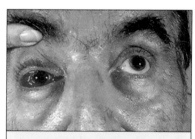

Fig. 211 Orbital cellulitis with chemosis and ophthalmoplegia, causing inability to look up.

Idiopathic orbital inflammatory syndrome, also known as orbital pseudotumor (Fig. 213), is a non-specific inflammation of the orbit with no identifiable local or systemic cause. It is the third most common orbital disorder behind thyroid and lymphoproliferative disease (see Fig. 215). An extensive rule-out workup often includes biopsy. Only then may oral, parental, or intralesional steroids be administered.

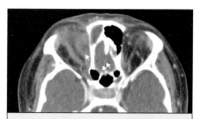

Fig. 212 CT scan of orbital cellulitis (↑) caused by ethmoid sinusitis (↑↑). Courtesy of Rand Kirtland, MD.

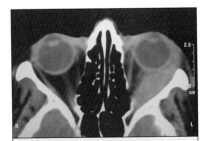

Fig. 213 MRI of left orbital pseudotumor, which is non-infectious inflammation of the orbit. Courtesy of Egal Leibovich, MD, and *Arch. Ophthalmol.*, 2007, Vol. 125, No. 12, pp. 1647–1651. Copyright 2007, American Medical Association. All rights reserved.

Exophthalmos

Exophthalmos (proptosis) is a protrusion of the eyeball caused by an increase in orbital contents. It is measured with an exophthalmometer (Fig. 214). In adults, unilateral and bilateral cases are most often due to thyroid disease. In children, unilateral cases are most often due to orbital cellulitis. Other causes are metastatic tumors, orbital hemorrhage, cavernous sinus thrombosis or fistulas, sinus mucoceles, orbital pseudotumor (Fig. 213), or the following primary orbital tumors:

1 hemangioma,
2 rhabdomyosarcoma,
3 lipoma,
4 dermoid,
5 lacrimal gland tumor,
6 glioma of the optic nerve,
7 lymphoma (Fig. 215),
8 meningioma (Fig. 118).

Enophthalmos

Enophthalmos is a retracted globe. The most common cause is a blow to the orbit that raises intraorbital pressure, causing the thin roof of the maxillary sinus to fracture (Fig. 216). This is called a "blow-out" fracture. Associated signs may include subconjunctival hemorrhage; entrapment of the inferior

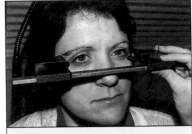

Fig. 214 Exophthalmometer.

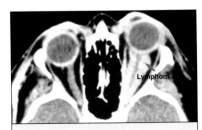

Fig. 215 CT scan of orbital lymphoma.

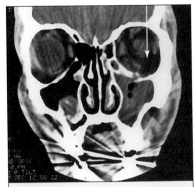

Fig. 216 CT scan of an orbital blow-out fracture (↓).

rectus muscle in the fracture causing restriction of upward gaze; and vertical diplopia (Fig. 217). Decreased sensation (hypesthesia) of the cheek is due to infraorbital nerve damage (Fig. 218). If diplopia or enophthalmos persist, or if more than 50% of the floor is blown out, a silicone, polyethylene, or titanium mesh may be placed under the eye.

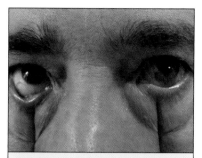

Fig. 218 Test for hypesthesia using two paper clips to compare the sensitivity on each side.

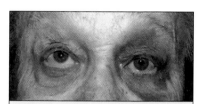

Fig. 217 Restriction of upward gaze due to blow-out fracture.

Chapter 6
Slit lamp examination and glaucoma

The slit lamp projects a beam of variable intensity onto the eye, which is viewed through a microscope (Fig. 219). The long, wide beam is useful in scanning surfaces such as lids, conjunctiva, and sclera. The long, narrow beam is for cross-sectional views (Figs 220 and 221). The short, narrow, intense beam is used to study cellular details (Fig. 363).

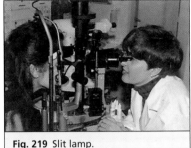

Fig. 219 Slit lamp.

Cornea

The cornea is the transparent, anterior continuation of the sclera devoid of both blood and lymphatic vessels. The grey corneoscleral junction is called the limbus. A slit beam cross-section of a normal cornea reveals the following as shown in Figs 221, 222, and 223A:

1 anterior band: epithelium on Bowman's membrane;
2 cross-section: through stroma;
3 posterior band: endothelium on Descemet's membrane.

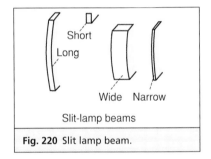

Slit-lamp beams

Fig. 220 Slit lamp beam.

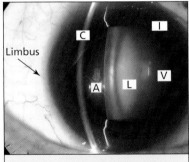

Fig. 221 Slit lamp view of anterior segment. C, cornea; A, anterior chamber; I, iris; L, lens; V, vitreous. Courtesy of Takashi Fujikado, MD.

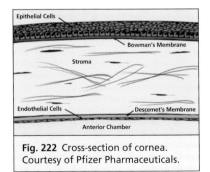

Fig. 222 Cross-section of cornea. Courtesy of Pfizer Pharmaceuticals.

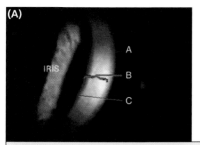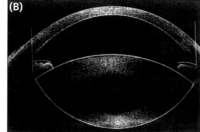

Fig. 223 (A) Slit beam cross-section of a cornea. A, epithelium; B, stroma; C, endothelium. (B) Tomogram of anterior segment showing thickness of cornea greatest in periphery. Courtesy of Richard Witlin, MD.

The corneal epithelium is the superficial covering of the cornea that is four to six layers thick and sits on Bowman's membrane. Its cells regenerate quickly so that 40% of the surface can regenerate in 24 hours. New cells are generated in the deepest layer sitting on Bowman's membrane and move toward the surface. The epithelial cells are also formed from the embryonic stem cells in the limbus (corneoscleral junction) and migrate across the cornea.

The stroma is the clear connective tissue layer and is thinnest in the center of the cornea (545 μm). It is almost twice as thick near the limbus (Fig. 223B). It contains the most densely packed number of sensory fibers in the body, 400 times that of skin. Abrasions and inflammations (keratitis) are, therefore, very painful. "Kerato" is a prefix that refers to cornea.

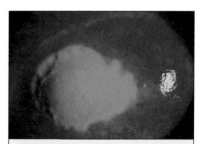

Fig. 224 Corneal abrasion stained with fluorescein.

The deepest endothelial layer sits on Descemet's membrane and is only one cell thick and doesn't regenerate. Its function is to pump fluid out of the cornea to maintain clarity.

Corneal epithelial disease

Commonly occurring epithelial abrasions (Figs 224 and 225), due to trauma, present with pain and a "red" eye. The de-epithelialized area stains bright green with fluorescein and a cobalt blue light. Rx:

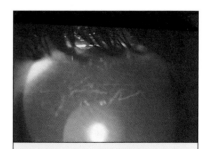

Fig. 225 Linear abrasions from trichiasis or particle under lid.

topical antibiotic, a cycloplegic (Cyclogel 1%), and an oral analgesic, with a pressure patch (two patches). Most abrasions clear quickly, within 24–48 hours, largely due to adjacent epithelial cells sliding over the abraded area.

To facilitate the examination of painful eyes, anesthetize with topical proparacaine 0.5%. It acts in seconds and lasts a few minutes. Never prescribe it for relief of pain because continued use damages the cornea.

Rarely, chemical or surgical trauma to the surface is so severe it destroys a large area of the limbus. In these cases, the epithelium cannot regenerate properly and a limbal cell transplant has to be done. Normal limbal tissue from the patient's other eye (autograft), from a relative (allograft) (Fig. 226), or from a cadaver may be used.

Corneal foreign bodies (Fig. 227) are removed with a sterile needle after placing two drops of proparacaine. Antibiotic drops are then prescribed.

Axenfeld nerve loops are intrascleral nerves that commonly appear normally as grey nodules under the bulbar conjunctiva (Fig. 228). Patients with a gritty sensation may confuse them with a foreign body and irritate the eyes further by trying to remove.

Localized epithelial edema (Fig. 229) has a translucent appearance, unlike an ulcer, which is opaque. In the common condition called recurrent corneal erosion, a small patch of edema develops where the epithelium does not adhere well to Bowman's membrane. This

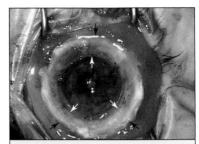

Fig. 226 A 360° limbal stem cell allograft: sutured or glued to sclera (↑). Courtesy of Clara Chan, MD, and Edward J. Holland, MD, Cincinnati Eye Institute.

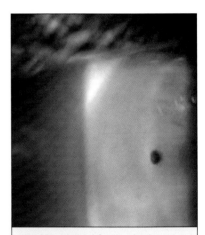

Fig. 227 Corneal foreign body. Courtesy of University of Iowa, Eyerounds.org.

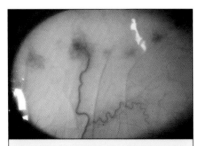

Fig. 228 Axenfeld loop. Courtesy of University of Iowa, Eyerounds.org.

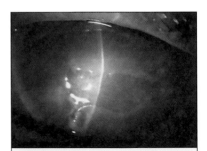

Fig. 229 Recurrent corneal erosion with localized epithelial edema.

often follows injury, but may be spontaneous. Patients awake in the morning with pain when cells slough off, usually just below the center of the cornea. The abrasion is treated with a patch and an antibiotic. The edematous epithelium is treated with hypertonic 2% or 5% sodium chloride solution (Muro 128) in the daytime and sodium chloride 5% ophthalmic ointment (Muro 128 ointment) at bedtime. If sloughing continues, roughing up Bowman's membrane with a needle (stromal puncture) increases adhesiveness of cells.

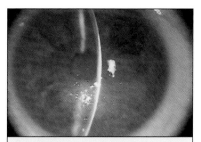

Fig. 230 Superficial punctate keratitis (SPK).

Superficial punctate keratitis (SPK) (Figs 230 and 234) is epithelial edema, which appears as punctate hazy areas that stain with fluorescein (Fig. 231). Burning, pain, and conjunctival redness may result, which is most common with dry eye. Inferior corneal edema occurs with an inability to close the lids, as occurs in Bell's palsy (Figs 105 and 106), lagophthalmos (Fig. 233), and with blepharitis of lower lid due to local release of toxic secretions. Reduced corneal sensation following LASIK surgery and in diabetes (neurotrophic keratitis) may cause dry eye and epithelial edema.

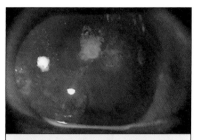

Fig. 231 SPK stained with fluorescein.

Filamentary keratitis is an irritating, light-sensitizing overgrowth of degenerated corneal epithelial cells. The strands of cells are often multiple and most often due to aging, dry eye, and trauma. They may be removed with a Nd:YAG laser (Fig. 232), but may recur. Prevent by treating underlying cause.

Corneal vascularization is a response to injury. Superficial vessels are most commonly a response to poorly fitting contact lenses

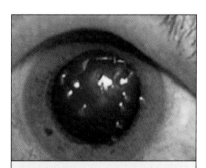

Fig. 232 Filamentary keratitis. Courtesy of University of Iowa, Eyerounds.org.

Superficial punctate keratitis (commonly causes photophobia)	
Traumatic causes	*Dessication*
Contact lenses	Dry eye due to decreased tear film production (see table, Chapter 4, Tear film)
Ultraviolet light	
Snow blindness	Dry eye resulting from increased evaporation due to:
Reaction from eye drops	
Chemical injury	1 inability to close lids after over-correction following blepharoplasty,
Blepharitis	
Trichiasis (Fig. 234)	2 CN VII nerve paralysis (Bell's palsy),
Rubbing eyes	3 thyroid exophthalmos.

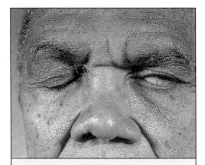

Fig. 233 Lagophthalmos is a condition in which the lids don't close completely.

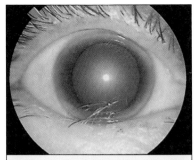

Fig. 234 SPK from trichiasis.

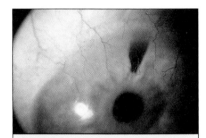

Fig. 235 Superficial vascularization, often due to poorly fitting contact lenses. Courtesy of Michael Kelly.

(Fig. 235), but also grow into areas damaged from ulcers, lacerations, or chemicals.

Chemical injuries with basic substances such as lye are most ominous because they immediately penetrate the depths of the cornea and permanently scar (Figs 236 and 237). Acid burns usually do not penetrate the stroma or scar. Rx: irrigate all chemical injuries immediately and profusely.

Epidemic keratoconjunctivitis (Fig. 238) is a common, highly infectious condition due to one of the adenoviruses that cause the common cold. There may be a severe conjunctivitis lasting up to 3 weeks associated with photophobia, fever, cold symptoms, and an adenopathy. The main problem is the keratitis, which can last for months or, rarely, years. It does not scar, but does restrict use of contact lenses until it clears. Wash your hands, instruments, chair, and door knobs especially well

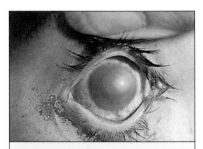

Fig. 236 Sodium hydroxide injury minutes after the event.

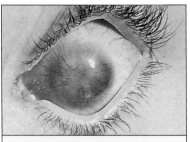

Fig. 237 Sodium hydroxide injury months after the event.

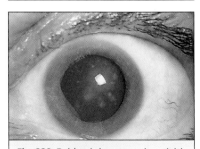

Fig. 238 Epidemic keratoconjunctivitis with characteristic white, punctate subepithelial infiltrates.

after evaluating this eye infection. Diluted povidone-iodine appears effective against virus in tears, but not replicating virus in cells. Topical steroid may relieve symptoms but prolongs the course.

Herpes simplex virus type 1 (HSV-1) is very common on the face, especially around the eyes and lips. At age 4, about 25% of the population are seropositive and this approaches 100% by age 60. When the corneal epithelium (Figs 239 and 240) is involved, the lesions, called dendrites, are similar in appearance to a branching tree, especially when stained with fluorescein. Diffuse punctate or round lesions can also occur. Patients complain of a gritty ocular sensation, conjunctivitis, and a history of a fever sore on the lip, nose, or mouth. Herpes often decreases corneal sensations. Compare the eyes by touching each with a cotton-tipped applicator, obviously testing the uninfected eye first. There may be small vesicles on the skin of the lids (Fig. 241). These often crust and then disappear within 3 weeks. The keratitis should be treated quickly because it can cause corneal opacities and loss of vision. When it penetrates the stroma, a chronic keratitis and iritis will require the cautious addition of topical steroids. Recurrences are common. Rx: generic trifluridine (Viroptic) 1% every 2 hours has been the mainstay treatment for years, but newly introduced Zirgan gel, ganciclovir 0.15%, can be used every 3 hours and is less toxic. Acyclovir 500 mg PO BID for 5 days may be added in resistant cases.

Anxious patients must be reassured that this eye disease is rarely due to HSV-2, which is a venereal disease transmitted by sexual contact.

Corneal ulcers are usually caused by a bacterial infection, although they occasionally be the result of a viral or fungal infection. They are characterized by conjunctivitis and a white patch of inflammatory cells in the cornea. Over 50% result from contact lens wear, especially lenses worn during sleep. Other causes include corneal abrasions, conjunctivitis, and blepharitis. Treat vigorously on an emergency basis, since it almost always scars and, in the case of *Pseudomonas*, may perforate within

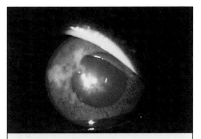

Fig. 239 Herpes simplex keratitis with tree-like branching lesions.

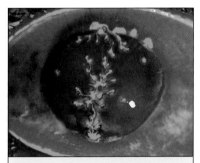

Fig. 240 Herpes simplex with large fluorescein-stained dendrites. Courtesy of Allan Connor, Princess Margaret Hospital, Toronto, Canada.

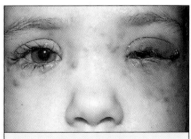

Fig. 241 Herpes dermatitis.

1 day (Fig. 244). Treatment often consists of more than one antibiotic drop and ointment (see table, Chapter 4, Common topical anti-infectives) with frequency of instillation dependent on severity and proximity to central visual axis.

Marginal ulcers (Fig. 242) are most common and may be due to infection or an immune reaction to staphyloccal toxins from associated chronic blepharitis. Rx: topical hourly broad-spectrum antibiotics. Steroids are sometimes used when a herpetic cause is confidently ruled out. Treat the blepharitis with lid scrubs, warm compresses, and massage of the lid margin.

Central ulcers (Fig. 243) are most ominous and in such cases cultures are always needed. Multiple topical broad-spectrum antibiotics are used up to every 15 minutes. The infection infrequently enters the globe (Fig. 243). When it does, a level of white cells may be seen in the anterior chamber, which is the space bounded anteriorly by the cornea and posteriorly by the iris and lens. This is called a hypopyon and might require a culture of the interior eye, especially if the vitreous is also involved.

Corneal endothelial disease

A monolayer of endothelial cells covers the deepest layer of the cornea and pumps fluid from the stroma to maintain corneal clarity. There are usually 2800 endothelial cells/mm², which do not replicate. When the number of cells drops below 500, or cells are damaged, corneal edema can occur and blurry vision and discomfort may result (Figs 245–247). The most common cause for this edema is cataract surgery. In these cases, the endothelial cells may be injured mechanically, chemically, or from rejection of the lens implant. This complication of cataract surgery is the most common reason leading to the need for corneal transplant surgery. Extremely elevated eye pressure (over 35 mmHg; Fig. 342), iritis, and a genetic weakness of the endothelium in Fuchs' dystrophy are also common causes. Very high pressure,

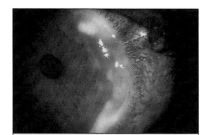

Fig. 242 Marginal corneal ulcer.

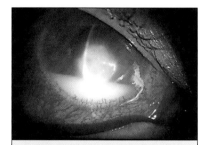

Fig. 243 Central corneal ulcer with secondary hypopyon.

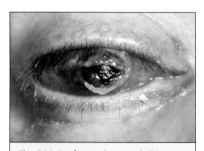

Fig. 244 Perforated corneal ulcer. Courtesy of Elliot Davidoff, MD.

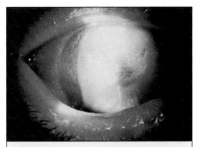

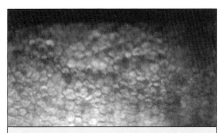

Fig. 245 Severe corneal edema with epithelial cysts is referred to as bullous keratopathy. It reduces vision and is usually very uncomfortable, often breaking down to painful corneal abrasions. Courtesy of Kenneth R. Kenyon, MD, and *Arch. Ophthalmol.*, Mar. 1976, Vol. 94, pp. 494–495.

Fig. 246 Specular microscopy of normal endothelial cell count, 2800 cells/mm², before cataract surgery.

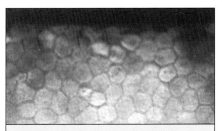

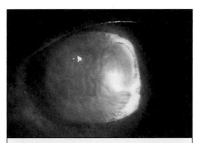

Fig. 247 Specular microscopy after cataract surgery that damaged the endothelium and caused corneal edema, resulting in a cell count of 680 cells/mm². If cells are damaged, they do not multiply to fill the gap. Instead, they enlarge and lose their normal hexagonal shape and their ability to pump fluid from the cornea. Courtesy of Martin Schneider, MD.

Fig. 248 Edematous folds in the cornea – called stria – usually result from low intraocular pressure. It is a similar effect to a balloon not fully blown up.

often over 40 mmHg in acute-angle glaucoma (Figs 335 and 336), temporarily damages the endothelium and causes corneal edema with the classic symptom of halos around lights. Symmetrel (amantadine), used to treat Parkinson's disease, could cause corneal edema by decreasing the endothelial cell count. Low pressure, below 5 mmHg, could also cause corneal cloudiness (Figs 248 and 324).

Fuchs' dystrophy is a genetic disorder of the Descemet's endothelial complex (Fig. 249) that results in drop out of endothelial cells. It is bilateral and is identified by guttata, which are

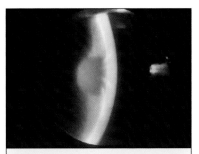

Fig. 249 Fuchs' dystrophy with central corneal thickening and haze due to edema. Courtesy of Hank Perry, MD.

small, round spots of thickening in Descemet's membrane. They are usually in the central corneal axis. It could lead to corneal edema and eventually require corneal transplant surgery.

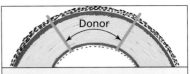

Fig. 250 Diagram outlining full-thickness corneal transplant (penetrating keratoplasty).

Corneal transplantation (keratoplasty)

Keratoplasty is one of the most successful organ transplant surgeries with more than a 90% success rate at 1 year and 80% after 10 years. In 2014, 46,500 procedures were performed in the USA using donor corneas from eye banks. Penetrating keratoplasty (Figs 250 and 251) – a full-thickness technique – is used to replace scarred, opacified stroma. Problems with penetrating keratoplasty are that it requires extensive suturing, which remains in place for over a year. It could take that amount of time for vision to return. Also, there is often a lot of residual astigmatism. For this reason, the newer technique, called Descemet-stripping endothelial keratoplasty (DSEK) (Figs 252–256) has now become the preferred procedure when there is no scarring of the stroma or other stromal disease such as keratoconus.

DSEK only replaces the endothelium, Descemet's membrane, and a tiny layer of stroma through a small wound. A third type of keratoplasty, called deep anterior lamellar keratoplasty (DALK), is done less frequently (1000 procedures/year) for eyes with

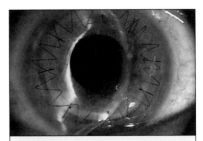

Fig. 251 Full-thickness corneal transplant (penetrating keratoplasty).

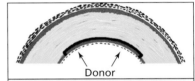

Fig. 252 DSEK: after removing damaged endothelium and Descemet's membrane, the donor tissue is folded to fit through a small wound. After unscrolling, an air bubble is injected to press the donor graft against the cornea. The endothelial cells' natural pumping action holds the graft in place without sutures.

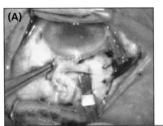
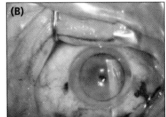

Fig. 253 Replacement of endothelium and Descemet's membrane. (A) Stripping of an 8.0 mm diameter of diseased endothelium and Descemet's membrane. (B) Insertion of folded donor graft. *Source:* Studeny Pavel, Farkis A. et al., *Br. J. Ophthalmol.*, 2010, Vol. 94, No 7. Reproduced with permission of BMJ Publishing Group, Ltd.

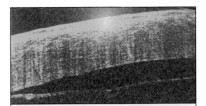

Fig. 254 OCT showing detached endothelial graft. Courtesy of Amar Agarwal, MD.

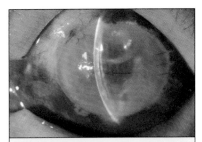

Fig. 255 DSEK graft separation (↑) 3 days after transplant. It was reattached by injecting an air bubble. Courtesy of Christopher Rapuano, MD, Wills Eye Hospital.

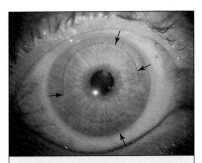

Fig. 256 Successful DSEK surgery with implant in place (↑). Courtesy of Henry Perry, MD.

stromal opacities and healthy endothelium (Figs 257–261). In DALK, just the anterior cornea is replaced, leaving behind a significant amount of posterior stroma with the endothelium and Descemet's membrane. Its advantage is that it can remove anterior corneal opacities, leaving behind the patient's own endothelial cells. The advantage of DALK is that immunologic rejection of donor endothelial cells is the leading cause of corneal graft failure.

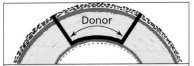

Fig. 257 DALK removes most of the stroma up to Descemet's membrane. A common complication is damage to the remaining thin, 10 μm layer. This complication necessitates converting to a penetrating keratoplasty 20% of the time.

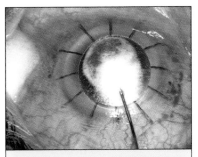

Fig. 258 DALK: step 1 is to inject air into the corneal stroma to begin separation of stroma from Descemet's membrane.

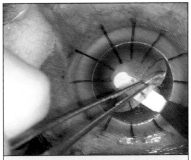

Fig. 259 DALK: step 2 is to complete stromal dissection with crescent blade.

A human corneal donor graft may be repeatedly rejected for immune reasons or because of a poor surface environment, as with dry eye or with a vascularized cornea that occurs with chemical burns (Figs 236 and 237). A last effort at maintaining clarity in the central axis is implantation of a graft utilizing a centrally located plastic lens. In 2007, 639 grafts of the Boston type were performed (Figs 262 and 263). Retroprosthetic membranes and glaucoma are more common complications.

Keratoconus (Figs 264–266) is a bilateral central thinning and bulging (ectasia) of the cornea to a conical shape with possible scarring. It is due to weakening of the stromal collagen. There may be an orange epithelial deposition of iron around the base of the cone called Fleischer's ring. It begins between ages 10 and 30, often in allergic persons. Rubbing the eye may cause or worsen the condition and should be discouraged. Once keratoconus is identified, topical anti-allergic medications and lubricants should be prescribed to eliminate rubbing. There is a higher incidence within families.

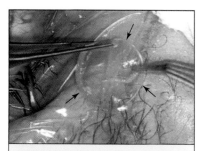

Fig. 260 DALK: step 3 is to remove Descemet's membrane from the donor cornea (↑).

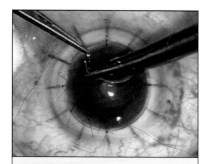

Fig. 261 DALK: step 4 is to suture donor graft to recipient bed. *Source:* D.C.Y. Han et al., *Am. J. Ophthalmol.,* 2009, Vol. 148(5), pp. 744–751. Reproduced permission of Elsevier.

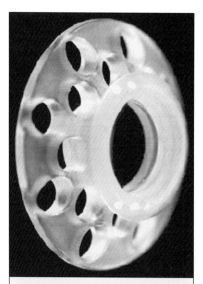

Fig. 262 The Boston Keratoprosthesis: collar-button device made of PMMA plastic. It is incorporated into a corneal graft that serves as carrier which is sutured in place like a standard graft.

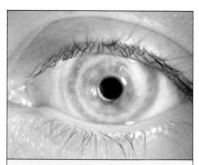

Fig. 263 Eye of a 23 year-old patient with congenital endothelial dystrophy. Four standard corneal grafts had failed. A Boston Keratoprosthesis implanted 5 years earlier resulted in consistent vision of 20/30 and normal pressure. Courtesy of Claes Dohlman, MD, PhD.

The resulting irregular type of astigmatism corrects poorly with glasses and may need soft or gas-permeable contact lenses to obtain clearer vision.

If the cornea continues to steepen, one may try to flatten it with intracorneal rings (Fig. 68) or chemically strengthen the stromal collagen using a new technique called cross-linking. In this procedure, riboflavin 0.1% solution is continuously dropped onto the cornea while the eye is irradiated with UVA light for

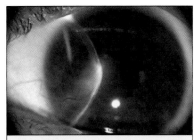

Fig. 264 Keratoconus with scarring at apex of cone.

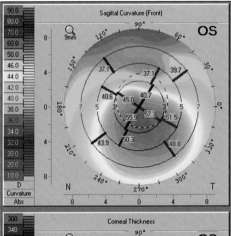

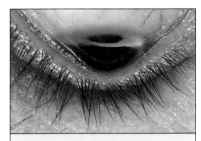

Fig. 265 Munson's sign: conical cornea indents lid when looking down. Courtesy of Michael P. Kelly.

Fig. 266 Corneal tomography of keratoconus showing thin, steep, eccentrically located corneal apex having a 57.3 D power with a thickness of only 449 μm. Normal central cornea averages 43 D with a thickness of 545 μm. Also diagnostic of keratoconus is a posterior corneal surface that is more steep (conical) than the anterior surface. Courtesy of Richard Witlin, MD.

30 minutes. It should only be used in cases of documented progression of disease. Severe keratoconus is treated with penetrating keratoplasty and accounts for 20% of corneal transplantation in the USA.

Down's syndrome occurs in about 1 in 800 births and is due to trisomy of chromosome 21. It is characterized by mental retardation, short stature, and a transverse palmar crease ("simian crease"). There is an increased incidence of keratoconus, strabismus, cataracts, and refractive errors (Fig. 267).

Argyrosis results from long-term exposure to topical or systemic silver (Fig. 268). Silver nitrate 2% eye drops were used extensively as an anti-infective in the first half of the twentieth century. It was the mainstay prophylactic therapy in newborns. Before its discovery in 1881 by Carl Crede 1 in 300 newborns were blinded by ophthalmia neonatorium. Erythromicin ointment has now replaced it in the delivery room.

Wilson's disease (hepatolenticular degeneration) is characterized by excessive deposition of copper in the liver and brain. It is a rare autosomal recessive disorder that often begins before age 40. The plasma copper-carrying protein – serum ceruloplasmin – is low. The pathognomonic sign of the condition is the brownish or grey-green Kayser–Fleischer ring (Fig. 269) due to copper depos-

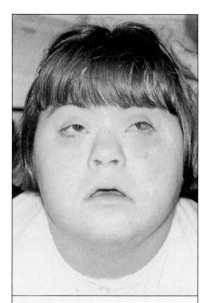

Fig. 267 Down's syndrome patient with keratoconus. Corneal edema (hydrops) is caused by a tear in Descemet's membrane. Also, note the characteristic flat face, small nose, low nasal bridge, narrow interpupillary distance, and upward slanting palpebral fissures. Courtesy of Kenneth R. Kenyon, MD, and *Arch. Ophthalmol.*, Mar. 1976, Vol. 94, pp. 494–495, Copyright 1976, American Medical Association., All rights reserved.

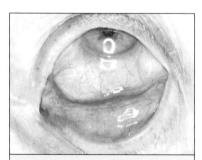

Fig. 268 Argyrosis: deposition of silver in conjunctiva, cornea, and lid. Silver nitrate eye drops were used in the past as a prophylactic antibacterial in newborns. Courtesy of Elliott Davidoff, MD.

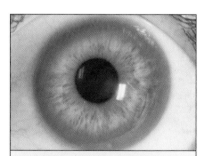

Fig. 269 Copper deposited in Descemet's membrane causing an orange ring at the limbus (Kayser–Fleischer ring) pathognomonic of Wilson's disease. Compare with corneal arcus shown in Appendix 1, Fig. 550. Courtesy of Denise de Freitas, MD. Paulista School of Medicine, Sao Paulo, Brazil.

its in Descemet's membrane, adjacent to the limbus.

Dermoid tumors (Fig. 270) are benign congenital growths often having protruding hairs. They are most common at the corneal limbus or in the orbit and may grow during puberty. They are removed if vision is threatened, or for discomfort and cosmetic reasons.

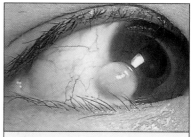

Fig. 270 Corneal dermoid.

Conjunctiva

The conjunctiva is a mucous membrane. The bulbar conjunctiva covers the sclera and ends at the corneal limbus. The palpebral conjunctiva lines the lids (Fig. 271). Fluid within the conjunctiva is called chemosis (Fig. 272) and is commonly seen in allergy, but also in infectious conjunctivitis, Grave's disease, and in rare cases of orbital venous congestion.

To examine the inner surface of the upper lid, first warn the patient, then "flip the lid" as follows:

1 have the patient look down with eyes open,
2 grasp eyelashes of upper lid at their bases,
3 pull out and up on lashes while pushing in and down on upper tarsal margin (patient should continue to look down during examination),
4 to return lid to normal position, have the patient look up.

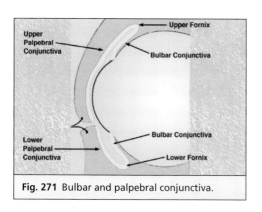

Fig. 271 Bulbar and palpebral conjunctiva.

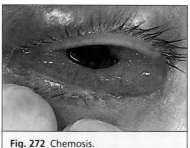

Fig. 272 Chemosis.

A pterygium (Figs 273–275) is a triangular growth of vascularized conjunctiva encroaching on the nasal cornea. Two causes are wind and ultraviolet light. It may be excised for cosmetic, comfort, or visual reasons. Recurrences of up to 30–40% are reported, but are significantly reduced to 2% by replacing excised conjunctiva with autograft (Figs 273–275).

A pinguecula (Figs 276 and 277) is a common, benign, yellowish elevation of the 180° conjunctiva, usually nasal, but also temporal. It is composed of collagen and elastic tissue. It occasionally becomes red, especially with allergies, and, rarely, may be removed if it is chronically inflamed, if it interferes with contact lens wear, or if it is a cosmetic problem.

Subconjunctival hemorrhages (Fig. 278) may be spontaneous. Common causes include rubbing of the eye or valsalva maneuvers, as occurs with coughing, sneezing, constipation, and heavy lifting. Elevated blood pressure and anticoagulants may increase the incidence.

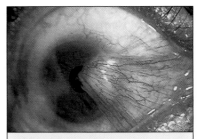

Fig. 273 Pterygium.

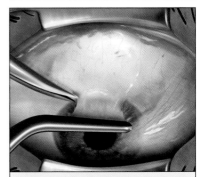

Fig. 274 Excision of conjunctival autograft from superior bulbar conjunctiva.

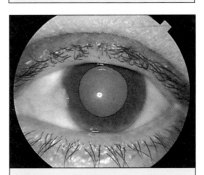

Fig. 276 Pinguecula.

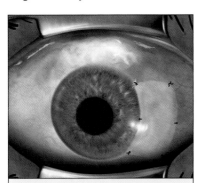

Fig. 275 Autograft is usually sutured (rarely glued) to nasal bulbar conjunctiva after removal of pterygium.

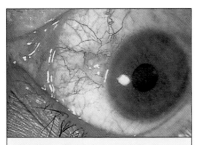

Fig. 277 Inflamed pinguecula.

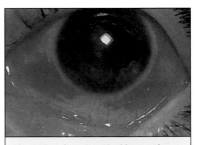

Fig. 278 Subconjunctival hemorrhage.

Lymphangiectasia refers to the engorgement of conjunctival lymphatic channels, most notably on the bulbar conjunctiva (Fig. 279). It is usually benign with no apparent cause. When symptomatic, it may be cauterized or excised.

Conjunctival concretions are commonly occurring, often multiple, small, benign, hard yellowish-white deposits of inspissated degenerative matter buried under the superficial palpebral conjunctiva (Fig. 280). They are usually asymptomatic unless the overlying conjunctiva erodes, at which time they cause a gritty sensation. They may be removed at the slit lamp with a topical anesthetic and sterile needle.

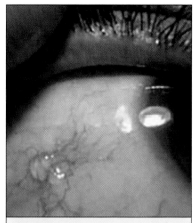

Fig. 279 Lymphangiectasia. Courtesy of University of Iowa, Eyerounds.org.

Conjunctival verruca (papilloma) is a benign neoplasm initiated after infection by human papillomavirus (Fig. 281). A symblepharon (Figs 10 and 283) is an adhesion of the bulbar and palpebral conjunctiva. Contracture can lead to an entropion with trichiasis. It is most commonly due to chemical burns, trachoma, epidemic keratoconjunctivitis, and the two following immune blistering mucocutaneous diseases.

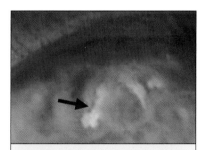

Fig. 280 Conjunctival concretions. Courtesy of University of Iowa, Eyerounds.org.

1 Stevens–Johnson syndrome, which is an acute blistering immune reaction to a foreign antigen, usually a drug (Fig. 10). It can affect the skin and/or the eyes and could be fatal.
2 Bullous pemphigoid (Fig. 282) is an autoimmune condition involving the skin and conjunctiva. It could last for years, and unlike Stevens–Johnson, it is not fatal. It is also confirmed by biopsy. Pemphix is Latin for blister.

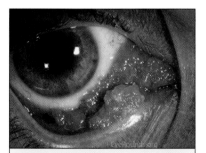

Fig. 281 Conjunctival verruca (wart) with typical cauliflower appearance. Courtesy of University of Iowa, Eyerounds.org.

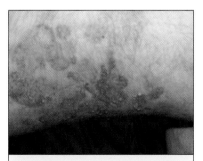

Fig. 282 Bullous pemphigoid causes conjunctivitis and itchy, red blisters on the skin.

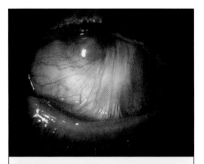

Fig. 283 Symblepharon: adhesions of bulbar to palpebral conjunctiva should be lysed with a glass rod or wet cotton applicator to prevent permanent scar. *Source*: Kheirkhah et al., *Am. J. Ophthalmol.*, 2008, Vol. 146, p. 271. Reproduced with permission of Elsevier.

Conjunctivitis causes redness with a gritty sensation. Common causes are tired eyes, pollutants, wind, dust, allergy, or infection (Fig. 284). If there is pain, it usually indicates corneal or intraocular involvement. Vascularized elevations of the palpebral conjunctiva, called papillae (Fig. 285), are a reaction to an inflamed eye. They are most unique to giant papillary conjunctivitis and vernal conjunctivitis.

Giant papillary conjunctivitis (or GPC) is a common cause for rejecting soft contact lenses. Large papillae develop under the lids. They are an immune reaction, usually in response to mucous debris on the lenses, and are more common in allergic individuals. Rx: change to a contact lens that is disposed of more frequently, i.e., every 2 weeks or even on a daily schedule; decrease wearing time; keep lenses especially clean; and sometimes discontinue lens wear.

Vernal conjunctivitis is an allergic condition in which large papillae are under the upper lid. They could abrade the cornea. It occurs in the first decade and may last for years. Both giant papillary conjunctivitis and vernal conjunctivitis may be treated with a topical mast cell inhibitor such as Cromolyn 4%

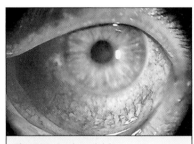

Fig. 284 Conjunctivitis.

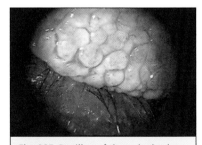

Fig. 285 Papillae of the palpebral conjunctiva.

solution. Sometimes steroid drops are also needed.

White lymphoid elevations of the conjunctiva (Fig. 286), called follicles, occur as a reaction to conjunctival irritation, especially from viruses, *Chlamydia*, and drugs.

1 Trachoma is a severe keratoconjunctivitis due to an infection by *Chlamydia trachomatis*. It affects 146 million people worldwide and is responsible for blindness in 6 million people outside the USA. It begins with papillae and follicles on the superior palpebral conjunctiva. Conjunctival shortening may result in an entropion, which causes trichiasis. Inflammation of the cornea leads to superior vascularization (pannus), occasional corneal scarring, and loss of vision (Fig. 287). Rx: a single dose of azithromycin, 20 mg/kg.

2 Inclusion conjunctivitis in adults is a follicular conjunctivitis (Fig. 286) with occasional keratitis. It is also due to *Chlamydia trachomatis* of a different serotype than that causing trachoma. This organism is the most common sexually transmitted pathogen and is the primary notifiable disease to the US Centers for Disease Control and Prevention. Its incidence rose in 2014, with 1,441,789 cases reported. Reported syphilis and gonorrhea also increased in 2014 with the latter being the second most reported pathogen. It is the most common cause of conjunctivitis in newborns, who acquire it passing through the birth canal in spite of the fact that erythromycin ointment is routinely given to newborns in the USA. Confirm with smear or culture by a gynecologist. Rx: oral doxycycline, tetracycline, or azithromycin and erythromycin ophthalmic ointment. Treat sexual partners.

Bacterial conjunctivitis has a white-yellow discharge and is often due to *Staphylococcus aureus*, *Streptococcus pneumonia*, and *Haemophilus influenzae*. It is usually treated without cultures (Figs 288 and 289) with inexpensive generic medications (see table, p. 59, Common topical anti-infectives). Ointments blur vision and are most useful for bedtime use. Erythromycin ointment is placed in the

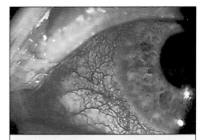

Fig. 286 Follicles of the palpebral conjunctiva.

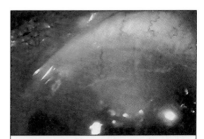

Fig. 287 Corneal inflammation from trachoma.

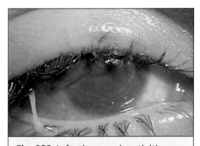

Fig. 288 Infectious conjunctivitis.

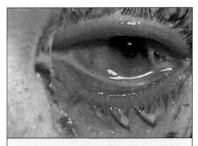

Fig. 289 Bacterial blepharoconjunctivitis.

eyes of most newborns to prevent chlamydial and other causes of conjunctivitis that might be picked up passing through the birth canal. Blepharitis should be suspected in cases of chronic recurring conjunctivitis, sties, and chalazia.

Viruses cause half the infectious cases of conjunctivitis. There is usually a watery discharge associated with "cold symptoms" and a swollen preauricular node. It is often treated with antibiotics since it is difficult to be sure the infection is not bacterial and cultures are not usually practical. Antibiotic/steroid combinations may relieve symptoms, but could aggravate an atypical herpes simplex infection.

Allergic conjunctivitis is a condition associated with intermittent itching, minimal conjunctival injection, stringy mucous discharge, chemosis, and puffy lids. Treatment begins with avoidance of known irritants, discontinuing make-up and applying cold compresses. When drops are needed, begin with over-the-counter drugs and then generic prescriptions, since they are less expensive and very effective. Expense of over-the-counter drugs: decongestants $7, decongestant/antihistamine $8, and antihistamine/mast cell stabilizer $13. Prescription drops range from $40 to $100.

A combination antihistamine/vasoconstrictor (pheniramine maleate/naphazoline) will often relieve discomfort and redness. The market cliché of "gets the red out" is true, but decongestants such as naphazoline and tetrahydrazoline have the undesireable effect of rebound hyperemia when discontinued. These drugs also dilate the pupil and could, rarely, cause attack of angle-closure glaucoma. Caution the patient to call an eye doctor if they experience eye pain, blurry vision, or increased redness. Ketotifen 0.025% (Zaditor or Alaway) is one of a group of over-the-counter drugs that stabilize mast cells, preventing histamine release. Fewer side effects make them safer for long-term use. Prescribe one drop twice a day. After trying antihistamines, decongestants, or mast cell stabilizers, one may try a NSAID that reduces the release of prostaglandin. Generic ketorolac 5% (Acular 5%) drops can be used QID PRN. Don't confuse ketorolac (a NSAID) with ketotifen (a mast cell stabilizer). If symptoms still persist, a steroid such as generic FML (fluorometholone 0.1%) solution or ointment may be added. Branded loteprednol 0.2% (Alrex) is another relatively safe steroid alternative.

When steroids are started, a slit lamp exam by an eye doctor is recommended because steroids could elevate eye pressure or precipitate a herpes simplex infection.

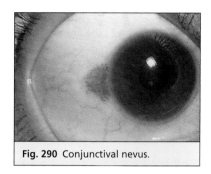

Fig. 290 Conjunctival nevus.

Oral antihistamines may be added. "Allergy shots" (immunotherapy) are usually reserved for more severe, chronic cases. After skin testing for sensitivity, an allergist may inject small amounts of the offending allergen over a 3–5 year period.

Conjunctival nevi (Fig. 290), often brown in color, are common. Malignant transformation of nevi to melanomas is rare. Malignant transformation is suggested by satellites, rapid growth, elevation, and inflammation (Fig. 291) and occurs 75% of the time from a pre-existing benign pigmented lesion.

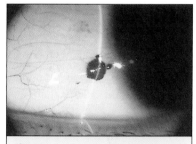

Fig. 291 Conjunctival melanoma.

Ocular melanosis oculi refers to hyperpigmentation of ocular structures including the iris, the choroid, and the trabecular meshwork, the latter of which may cause glaucoma. The episclera and sclera may appear slate blue (Fig. 292). When the skin is involved it is called oculodermal melanocytosis (nevus of Ota). This condition is associated with a high rate of melanoma and should be monitored.

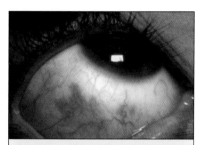

Fig. 292 Melanosis oculi. Courtesy of University of Iowa, Eyerounds.org.

Conjunctivitis			
	Viral	*Bacterial*	*Allergic*
Onset	Acute	Acute	Intermittent
Associated complaints	Often sore throat, rhinitis, fever	Often none	History of allergy; nasal or sinus stuffiness, dermatitis
Discharge	Watery	Thick, yellow	Stringy mucus
Preauricular node	Common	Infrequent	None

Sclera

The sclera is the white, fibrous, protective outer coating of the eye that is continuous with the cornea. The episclera is a thin layer of vascularized tissue that covers the sclera.

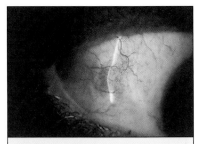

Fig. 293 Episcleritis has a 60% occurrence rate.

Episcleritis is a localized, elevated, and tender, but not usually painful, inflammation of the episclera (Fig. 293). It lasts for weeks and may be suppressed with topical steroid if itchy or uncomfortable. It is often a non-specific immune response but, infrequently, occurs in gout, syphilis, rheumatoid arthritis, and gastrointestinal disorders.

Scleritis is a severe inflammation of the sclera that may cause blindness. Unlike episcleritis, it is often painful. A quarter of the cases are associated with systemic immune or infectious diseases such as systemic lupus erythematosis, rheumatoid arthritis, Lyme disease, tuberculosis, and syphilis, to name a few. Anterior scleritis is associated with visible engorgement of vessels deep to the conjunctiva (Fig. 294). Posterior scleritis causes choroidal effusions and even retinal detachments. Systemic corticosteroids, antimetabolites, or anti-infective drugs are usually required. Blood tests may include angiotensin-converting enzyme (ACE) for sarcoidosis; antinuclear antibody (ANA) for lupus; c-antineutrophil cytoplasmic antibody (c-ANCA) for Wegener's granulomatosis; p-antineutrophil cytoplasmic antibody (p-ANCA) for arteritis; fluorescent treponemal antibody (FTA)-ABS and Venereal Disease Research Laboratory (VDRL) text for syphilis; ELISA Western blot for Lyme disease; rheumatoid factor (RF) for rheumatoid arthritis; and C-reactive protein and erthyrocyte sedimentation rate for non-specific systemic inflammation.

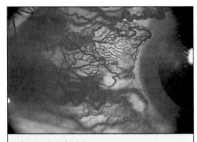

Fig. 294 Scleritis.

A blue sclera is due to increased scleral transparency, which allows choroidal pigment to be seen. It occurs normally in newborns, and abnormally in osteogenesis imperfecta (blue sclera with brittle bones), or following scleritis in rheumatoid arthritis (Fig. 295).

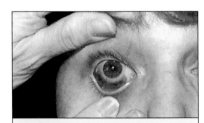

Fig. 295 Rheumatoid arthritis causing thin sclera with visible underlying choroid.

A staphyloma is a localized prolapse of bluish uveal tissue into thinned sclera. It occurs in rheumatoid arthritis, pathologic myopia (often over 10 D), or trauma (Fig. 296).

Jaundice, or icterus, refers to yellowing of the skin or sclera due to increased levels of bilirubin (Fig. 297). Because the elastin in the sclera has an increased affinity for bilirubin, it is often the first symptom of the condition. Total bilirubin is usually 0.3–1.0 mg/dL in adults and 1.0–12 mg/dL in newborns. Icterus first becomes toxic in adults above 12 mg/dL. Above this level, newborns could develop mental retardation; a condition called kernicterus.

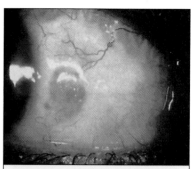

Fig. 296 Staphyloma is a weakening of the sclera causing a bulging of the wall of the eye (ectasia). It is most often due to pathologic myopia, trauma, elevated eye pressure, or inflammatory damage from scleritis.

Glaucoma

Glaucoma is a disease of the optic nerve due to elevated intraocular pressure pressing on the blood supply to the nerve or on the ganglion cell axon disrupting axonal transport (see Fig. 310).

Intraocular pressure is maintained by a balance between aqueous inflow and outflow. The aqueous produced by the ciliary body passes from the posterior chamber (the space behind the iris) through the pupil into the anterior chamber (Figs 298–300). It then drains through the trabecular meshwork through the venous canal of Schlemm and exits the eye through the episcleral veins.

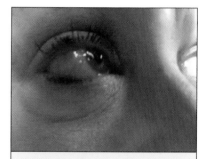

Fig. 297 Jaundice (icterus): yellow skin and sclera due to elevated bilirubin.

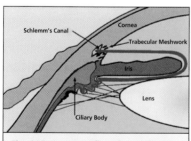

Fig. 298 Aqueous flow from ciliary body to Schlemm's canal. Courtesy of Pfizer Pharmaceuticals.

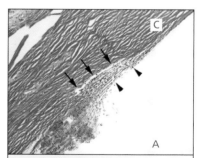

Fig. 299 Histology showing Schlemm's canal (arrows), trabecular meshwork (arrowheads), aqueous (A), and cornea (C).

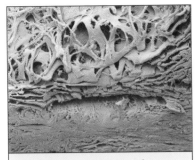

Fig. 300 Microscopic view of trabecular meshwork.

Glaucoma vs. glaucoma suspect

Normal intraocular pressure is 10–20 mmHg and should be measured at different times of day as there is a diurnal rhythm. Pressure greater than 28 mmHg is usually treated regardless of other findings. Treat pressures of 20–27 mmHg when there is loss of vision, a family history of glaucoma, damage to the optic nerve as evidenced by disk palor with cupping, thinning of the nerve fiber layer as shown on OCT testing, and/or GDx scanning polarimetry (see Figs 314–317, below). Patients with pressures of 20–27 mmHg without other suspicious findings of glaucoma are called glaucoma suspects. They are followed with more frequent visits than usual, with monitoring of visual fields and optic nerve changes. When treatment is started pressures are usually kept below 20 mmHg, which most often prevents loss in vision. However, some patients may lose vision even when pressures are kept in the high teens. These eyes require further lowering of pressure to the low teens and such patients have the condition referred to as low-pressure or normal-tension glaucoma. It is present in over 90% of Koreans and Japanese with glaucoma and in 50% of glaucoma patients worldwide.

Several instruments can be used to indirectly measure intraocular pressure by indenting the cornea, as follows.

1 A Goldmann applanation tonometer (Fig. 301) is the most accurate instrument for this purpose. It is used in conjunction with a slit lamp, and requires the use of anesthetic drops and fluorescein dye.

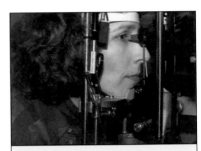

Fig. 301 Goldmann tonometer.

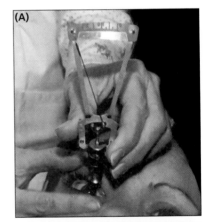

(A)

(B)

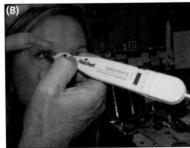

Fig. 302 (A) Schiötz tonometer. (B) Tono-Pen applanation tonometer.

2 The Schiötz tonometer and Tono-Pen are portable instruments (Fig. 302) that indent the anesthetized cornea and are used for bedside measurements.

3 The air-puff tonometer tests the pressure by blowing a puff of air at the eye. It is used by technicians since it does not require eye drops or corneal contact, but is more uncomfortable and slightly less accurate.

With all three instruments, the tonometric pressure reading is only an estimate of the real pressure. A thick cornea requires extra force to indent and, therefore, gives a falsely elevated reading, and the opposite is true with thin corneas. To better approximate the real pressure – especially in glaucoma suspects where exactitude is important – an ultrasonic pachymeter is used to measure corneal thickness. A conversion factor for corneal thickness then adjusts the tonometric reading upward with thin corneas or downward with thick corneas (Fig. 303).

The iridocorneal angle

Aqueous leaves the eye by entering the trabecular meshwork (Figs 299 and 304) which is the tan to dark brown band at the angle between the cornea and iris. It then exits the eye after entering the canal of Schlemm, which is a 360° circular tube leading into the scleral and episcleral venous plexus. The angle, normally 15–45°, can be estimated with a slit lamp (Figs 305 and 306), but a goniolens (Figs 307 and 308) is more accurate. In

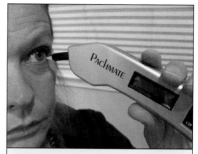

Fig. 303 Measurement of corneal thickness with ultrasonic pachymeter.

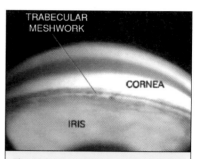

Fig. 304 Normal trabecular meshwork: grade 4 angle as seen in a goniolens.

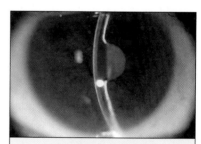

Fig. 305 Narrow angle in short hyperopic eye.

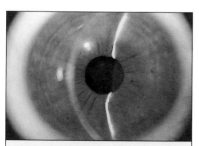

Fig. 306 Deep anterior chamber with wide open angle in long myopic eye.

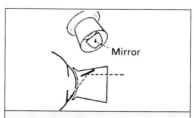

Fig. 307 Trabecular meshwork seen with a goniolens.

open-angle glaucoma, the trabecular mesh-work and the canal of Schlemm are obstruct-ed, whereas in narrow-angle glaucoma the space between the iris and cornea is too nar-row, so aqueous cannot reach the trabecular meshwork. A narrow angle at risk of closing is graded 0–2 (see Fig. 309). Angles of grade 3 or 4 are considered wide open with no chance of closing.

The optic disk (optic papilla)

The disk is the circular junction where the ganglion cell axons exit the eye, pick up a myelin sheath, and become the optic nerve (Figs 310–313). The lamina cribrosa is the per-forated continuation of the scleral wall of the eye that allows passage of the retina gangli-on cell axons and the central retinal artery

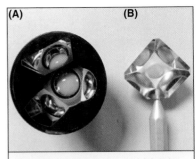

Fig. 308 (A) Goldmann and (B) Zeiss gonioscope lenses used to examine the angle of the eye at the slit lamp.

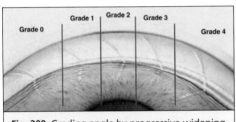

Fig. 309 Grading angle by progressive widening from 0 to 4. Courtesy of Pfizer Pharmaceuticals.

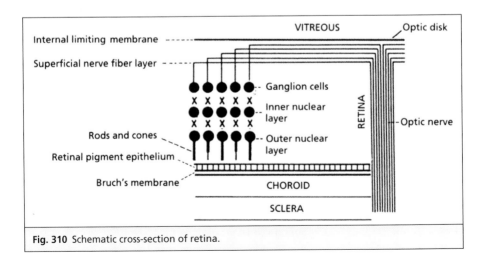

Fig. 310 Schematic cross-section of retina.

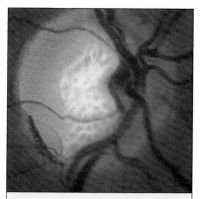

Fig. 311 Lamina cribrosa forms the floor of optic disk. Note perforations for passage of nerves and blood vessels. Courtesy of University of Iowa, Eyerounds.org.

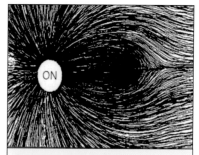

Fig. 312 Drawing of retinal nerve fiber layer with 1.2 million ganglion cell axons converging to make up the optic nerve (ON).

and veins to exit the globe (Fig. 316). It forms the bottom of the optic cup that is usually less than one-third the disk diameter, although larger cups can be normal.

Signs of nerve fiber damage
(Figs 312–317)

As pressure damages the nerve:

1 cup/disk ratio increases (Fig. 314),
2 cup becomes more excavated and often unequal in the two eyes,
3 vessels shift nasally,
4 disk margin loses capillaries and turns pale, with infrequent flame hemorrhage,
5 diffuse loss of retinal nerve fiber layer.

The optic disk changes can be followed by accurate drawings, photographs, or OCT or GDx testing (Figs 315–317).

Retinal nerve fiber layer thickness is usually measured around the optic disk (less often the macula) with OCT or GDx. It is most useful in detecting early stages of glaucoma before visual field loss becomes evident. A 5 μm progressive loss of thickness between tests is significant. (A red blood cell has a diameter of 7 μm.)

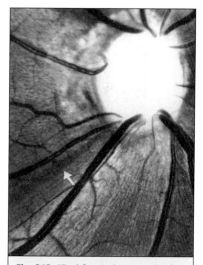

Fig. 313 "Red-free" photograph of glaucomatous cupping and loss of retinal nerve fiber layer (white arrow). The dark area with loss of striations is pathognomonic of fiber loss if it fans out and widens further from disk. Courtesy of Michael P. Kelly.

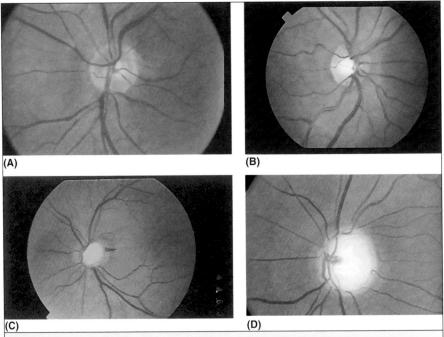

Fig. 314 Optic cup/disk ratio (A) C/D = 0.25; (B) C/D = 0.40; (C) C/D = 0.70 with hemorrhage; (D) C/D = 0.90.

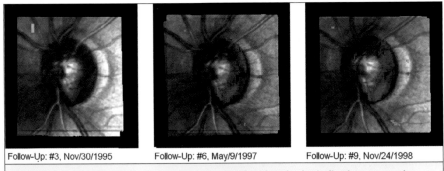

Follow-Up: #3, Nov/30/1995   Follow-Up: #6, May/9/1997   Follow-Up: #9, Nov/24/1998

Fig. 315 Scanning laser optic disk tomography (OCT) with red color indicating progressive cupping over 3 year period. Courtesy of Heidelberg Engineering, Inc.

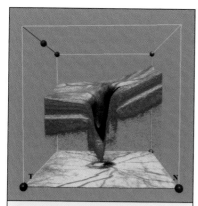

Fig. 316 Three-dimensional OCT using high-speed ultra-high resolution to create multiple cross-sectional images of optic nerve cupping. Courtesy of Elizabeth Affel, OCT-C, Wills Eye Hospital.

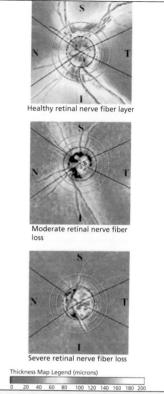

Healthy retinal nerve fiber layer

Moderate retinal nerve fiber loss

Severe retinal nerve fiber loss

Thickness Map Legend (microns)

0   20   40   60   80   100 120 140 160 180 200

Fig. 317 Color-coded GDx scanning laser polarimetry showing loss of thicker (yellow) nerve fiber layer over several years. It should be noted that the nerve fiber layer is normally thickest inferiorly then superiorly, followed by nasally, and then temporally. This can be rememberd by the acronym ISN'T. Courtesy of Carl Zeiss Meditec., Inc.

Visual field defects pathognomonic of glaucoma (Fig. 318)

1 Bjerrum's scotoma extends nasally from the blind spot in an arc.

2 Island defects could enlarge into a Bjerrum's scotoma.

3 Constricted fields occur before loss of central vision.

4 Ronne's nasal step is loss of peripheral nasal field above or below the horizontal.

The diagnosis and treatment of open-angle glaucoma should initially be made before visual field loss based on eye pressure, optic nerve findings, nerve fiber layer thickness, and family history. If one waits for visual field loss, 20% of the nerve fiber layer may have already been lost.

The goal is to reduce pressure below 20 mmHg, or at least to a level where there is no further loss of visual field or increase in cupping. Each patient should have a target pressure we try to attain. It is set at a lower pressure in severe glaucoma, or, if optic nerve damage continues to progress. Maintenance

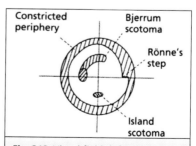

Fig. 318 Visual field defects in glaucoma.

of pressures in the high teens is usually sufficient. Continued progression of visual field loss and nerve fiber damage occurring with pressures controlled in the high teens requires further pressure lowering, often to the low teens. This is referred to as low-tension glaucoma. It may require a combination of medications, one from each of the classes in the table opposite, or the addition of a surgical procedure (Figs 319–334).

Before surgery, be sure the drops are being used properly. Only 20% of the eye drop is retained on the surface of the eye with most of it running onto the cheek or into the nose. Only half of the 20% remains in the eye after 4 minutes and only 3.4% remains after 10 minutes. Therefore, one should wait 10 minutes before administering a second drop. The effectiveness of a drop is increased by closing the eyelids and applying digital pressure to the punctal area (Fig. 143).

Unfortunately, up to 60% of patients are noncompliant in using their drops on schedule, especially when using more than one drop. Always ask whether drops were used before the present visit.

Surgical procedures for open-angle glaucoma

After being convinced that the patient is using the drops properly, and if they still do not control the pressure, surgery can be performed. Procedures are first directed at increasing aqueous outflow, or, less often, at reducing aqueous secretion. Argon laser trabeculoplasty or a technique called selective laser trabeculoplasty (SLT), both of which increase outflow, are often the first choice (Figs 319 and 320). The latter uses less energy and may be repeated. If pressure is still too high, a surgical hole is created at the limbus

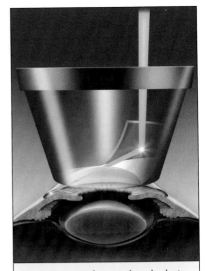

Fig. 319 Argon laser trabeculoplasty requires a reflecting mirror on the eye to visualize and focus the laser on the trabecular meshwork hidden from direct view.

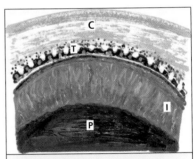

Fig. 320 Drawing of argon laser trabeculoplasty. Up to 100 burns (white discoloration) may be applied to the junction of the pigmented and non-pigmented trabecular meshwork around the entire 360° circumference. The pressure-lowering effect is likely due to the contraction of tissue around the trabecular meshwork stretching open the drainage pores. C, cornea; T, trabecular meshwork; I, iris; P, pupil.

Class and action	Chemical name	Trade name	Concentration	Dosage	Comment
Beta-blocker ↓ Aqueous secretion	Betaxolol (G)	Betoptic S	0.25% eye drops	BID	Slows heart rate Aggravates respiratory conditions
	Timolol (G, PF)	Timoptic, Betimol	0.25 & 0.5% eye drops	BID	Betoptic is cardioselective with the fewest systemic side effects
	Timoptic gel (G)	Timoptic XE	0.25 & 0.5% eye drops	QD	
Prostaglandin analogue ↑Aqueous outflow	Latanoprost (G)	Xalatan	0.005% eye drops	HS	Darkening and lengthening of of eyelashes, with hyperpigmentation of iris and periocular (eyelid) skin, loss of orbital fat (Figs 11–13). Also, iritis macular edema, and conjunctivitis
	Travoprost (G)	Travatan Z	0.004% eye drops		
	Bimatoprost	Lumigan	0.01 & 0.03% eye drops		
	Tafloprost (PF)	Zioptan	0.0015% eye drops		
Alpha-adrenergic agonist ↓Aqueous secretion ↑Aqueous outflow	Brimonidine (G)	Alphagan P 0.1%	0.01, 0.15, & 0.2% eye drops	TID	Frequent allergy
Carbonic anhydrase inhibitor					
Topical	Dorzolamide (G)	Trusopt	2% eye drops	TID	Could suppress bone marrow
	Brinzolamide	Azopt	1% eye drops	TID	
Oral ↓Aqueous secretion	Acetazolamide (G)	Diamox	250 & 500 mg tablet	250 mg, 500 mg	Could suppress bone marrow
Cholinergic ↑Aqueous outflow	Pilocarpine (G)	Pilocar	0.5–6.0% eye drops	QID	Retinal detachment, cataracts, small pupil, brow ache
Combination	Brimonodine and Brinzolamide	Simbrinza	0.2 & 1% eye drops	BID	Convenient
	Timolol and Dorzolomide (G, PF)	Cosopt	0.5 & 2% eye drops	BID	
	Brimonidine and Timolol	Combigan	0.2 & 0.5% eye drops		

Generic (G) or preservative-free (PF) available.

(trabeculectomy) to drain aqueous through the sclera and under the conjunctiva (Figs 321–325). The trabeculectomy could be repeated if the hole closes. If still unsuccessful, a tube could be implanted connecting the anterior chamber with the subconjunctival space (Fig. 326). These two methods expose the interior of the eye to infection since only the overlying conjunctiva protects the inner globe (Fig. 325). If the post-operative pressure is too low – usually less than 5 mmHg – the hypotony could cause permanent damage to the macula (Fig. 324). This often results from wound leaks. These leaks are identified with the Seidel test whereby a fluorescein strip is placed on the suspected site and cobalt-blue-filtered light used to show the stream of aqueous.

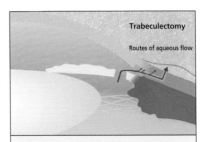

Fig. 321 Surgical trabeculectomy showing aqueous flow from ciliary body through iridectomy and scleral tunnel. It exits eye under conjunctiva. Courtesy of Pfizer Pharmaceuticals.

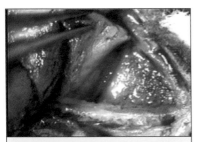

Fig. 322 The sclera is dissected toward the limbus to expose Schlemm's canal. Courtesy of iScience.

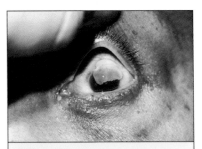

Fig. 323 A trabeculectomy is a surgically created fistula from anterior chamber to subconjunctival space. This bleb was too large and irritated the cornea and needs to be revised. Courtesy of Steven Brown, MD, and *Arch. Ophthalmol.*, Nov. 1999, Vol. 1, p. 156 Copyright 1999, American Medical Association. All rights reserved.

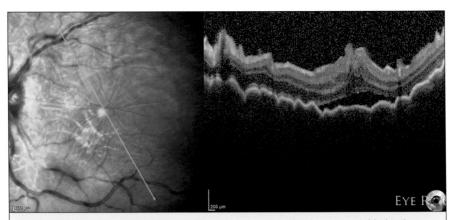

Fig. 324 Fundus photo with OCT scan of hypotony maculopathy showing wrinkled retina. A target pressure of 6 mmHg or more is usually sought. Courtesy of University of Iowa, Eyerounds.org.

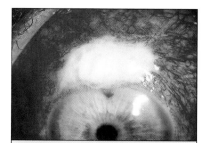

Fig. 325 The rate of trabeculectomy bleb-related infection is about 1.5% after 2 years, but is reported up to 8% when followed for longer periods. This conjunctival bleb was too thin and got infected. The interior of this eye is at risk of endophthalmitis, which could cause blindness. Courtesy of Donald L. Bendenz and *Arch. Ophthalmol.*, Aug. 1999, Vol. 117, p. 1010. Copyright 1999, American Medical Association. All rights reserved.

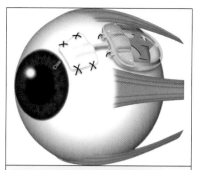

Fig. 326 Ahmed glaucoma valve. Tube in anterior chamber drains aqueous to subconjunctival space. Courtesy of New World Medical, Inc.

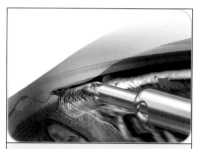
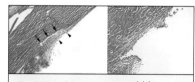

Fig. 327 Trabectome unroofing Schlemm's canal. Invented by Roy Chuck, MD, and George Baerveldt, MD, Albert Einstein Medical School.

Two new glaucoma surgeries have recently been introduced to increase aqueous outflow. Their advantage is that compared to trabeculectomy there is less risk of infection and hypotony since they do not depend on a thin conjunctival covering. One technique uses a surgical instrument called a trabectome. It uses electrical pulses to vaporize about 90° of diseased trabecular tissue that obstructs access to Schlemm's canal (Figs 327–329).

The other new procedure is called canaloplasty (Figs 330–332). In this technique a suture is placed in Schlemm's canal and is then tied and tightened to stretch it open. Neither of these techniques has yet replaced the gold standard of trabeculectomy.

Fig. 328 Schlemm's canal (↓↓↓), trabecular meshwork (↑↑).

The above-discussed surgeries increase aqueous outflow from the eye. Another strategy is to surgically reduce aqueous inflow by destroying some of the ciliary processes. To accomplish this, transscleral "cryo" or laser therapy may be applied to the area directly overlying the ciliary processes (Fig. 333) or endoscopic cyclophotocoagulation may be performed by entering the eye and destroying the ciliary process with direct visualization (Fig. 334).

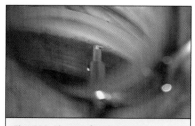

Fig. 329 Photo of trabectome.

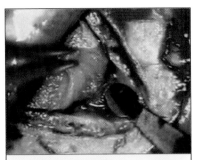

Fig. 330 Dissection of sclera towards the limbus. A window of the sclera is then removed for entry into Schlemm's canal.

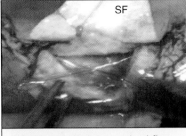

Fig. 331 Canaloplasty: a scleral flap (SF) is created to expose Schlemm's canal. A microcatheter is then threaded into Schlemm's canal. It is then withdrawn dragging a suture with it that remains in place.

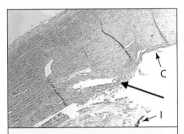

Fig. 332 Histology of the angle between the cornea (C) and the iris (I) showing suture in Schlemm's canal.

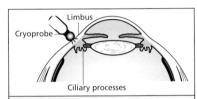

Fig. 333 Transscleral cryotherapy is applied for less than 20 seconds to 180° of sclera 1 mm posterior to the limbus. Transscleral diode laser may also be used to destroy part of the ciliary body.

Angle-closure glaucoma

Angle-closure glaucoma is less common than the previously discussed open-angle glaucoma and its treatment is different. It usually occurs in hyperopic eyes that are short with crowded anterior segments. The iris in these eyes is closer to the cornea (Figs 305–309). The resulting narrow angle becomes even more narrow when the pupil becomes mid-dilated. In this position, there is maximum contact between the iris and lens, preventing the aqueous from reaching the anterior chamber and trabecular meshwork. This "pupillary block" traps aqueous behind the iris and pushes the iris forward even more until the angle is totally closed. The total closure of the angle causes a sudden elevation in pressure, often exceeding 60 mmHg. This

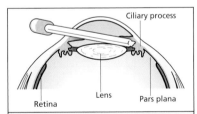

Fig. 334 Endoscopic cyclophotocoagulation for partial destruction of aqueous-secreting ciliary processes. One probe consisting of a light *source*, laser, and camera is usually inserted into the eye near the corneal limbus, although a pars plana site may be used. Anywhere from 170° to 280° is usually treated.

pressure damages the pupil, causing it to remain fixed and dilated.

Symptoms include pain, blurred vision, halos, and nausea. Signs include a mid-dilated non-reactive pupil, and corneal edema, with venous engorgement of conjunctival vessels (Figs 335 and 336).

Pupil dilation precipitating this attack may be caused by stimulation of the pupillary dilator muscle by adrenergic drugs, stress, or darkness. Anticholinergic drugs, such as major tranquilizers, block the sphincter muscle and may trigger an attack.

Treatment of angle-closure glaucoma first requires lowering of the pressure to break the attack and clear the cornea. It usually includes pilocarpine 1% to constrict the pupil and up to three other pressure-lowering types of eye drops. If the pressure still remains too high, a short-acting hyperosmotic agent such as intravenous mannitol 20% or oral glycerine 50% may be administered. Both draw fluid out of the eye by increasing the osmolarity of the blood. Once the attack is arrested, the corneal edema may be further cleared with topical hypertonic 2% saline solution. Then,

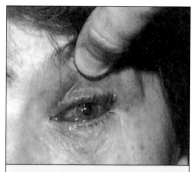

Fig. 335 Acute angle-closure glaucoma with dilated pupil.

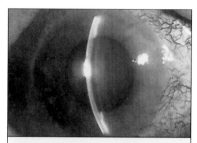

Fig. 336 Angle-closure glaucoma: shallow anterior chamber and corneal edema.

Common types of glaucoma		
	Primary open-angle glaucoma	*Angle-closure glaucoma*
Occurrence	70% of all glaucomas	10% of all glaucomas
Etiology	Unknown obstruction in trabecular meshwork, usually inherited; increases with age	Closed-angle glaucoma increases with age and hyperopia
Symptoms	Usually asymptomatic	Red, painful eye; halos around lights; nausea
Signs	Elevated pressure Increased disk cupping Visual field defect	Markedly elevated pressure Steamy cornea Fixed, mid-dilated pupil Conjunctival injection
Treatment	Usually eye drops	Laser iridotomy
Contraindicated medications	Corticosteroids: high doses or long-term use mandate pressure testing	Pupil dilators such as adrenergics, anticholinergics, antihistamines, major tranquilizers

a laser iridotomy can be performed (Fig. 337). This allows aqueous to flow into the anterior chamber and bypass the pupillary block. It is often a permanent cure and the pupil may then be safely dilated.

Less common types of glaucoma, called secondary open-angle glaucoma, could be caused by blockage of the trabecular meshwork by pigment (as in melanosis oculi) (Fig. 292 and 338), hemorrhage (Fig. 340), inflammatory cells (as in iritis), pseudoexfoliation (Fig. 339), scarring from rubeosis iridis (Figs 359 and 360) or venous congestion due to orbital disease and cavernous sinus thrombosis or fistula.

Trauma could cause glaucoma by tearing the iris at its insertion on the ciliary body. Gonioscopy may reveal angle recession (Fig. 341), in which the iris insertion is torn posteriorly, exposing a wide band of darkly pigmented ciliary body. Often, there is associated bleeding in the anterior chamber (Fig. 340), referred to as a hyphema. Complications of hyphema include rebleeds, associated retinal damage, and glaucoma. Rx: bilateral patch and absolute bedrest for 5 days. Patients should be monitored indefinitely because about 10% ultimately develop glaucoma.

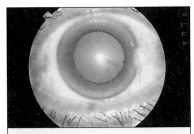

Fig. 337 Peripheral iridotomy at 2 o'clock.

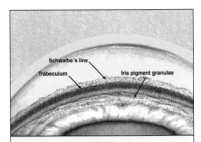

Fig. 338 Pigment of dispersion syndrome causing secondary glaucoma.

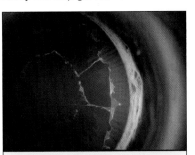

Fig. 339 Pseudoexfoliation is identified by white flakes on the anterior lens capsule, pupillary margin, zonules, and trabecular meshwork. It is relatively common and is associated with an increased incidence of glaucoma and weakened zonules which could complicate cataract surgery. Courtesy of Rhonda Curtis, CRA, COT, Washington University Medical School, St. Louis, MO, and *J. Ophthalmic Photogr.*

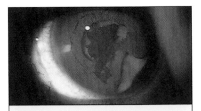

Fig. 340 Hyphema with large iris disinsertion (dialysis) from its root.

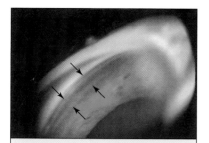

Fig. 341 Angle recessed posteriorly following traumatic hyphema. The recessed angle is seen as a wide, dark band between the cornea and the iris (↑).

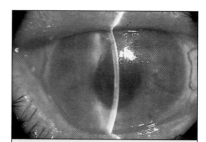

Fig. 342 Glaucoma causing a cloudy, edematous cornea.

Congenital glaucoma is fortunately rare, but must be suspected since routine office eye pressure measurements are difficult, if not impossible, in infants and young children. Clues to arouse suspicion are squinting, tearing, an enlarged globe (buphthalmos) (Fig. 343), and corneal edema. The latter may cause a subtle loss of a normally shiny, clear corneal surface (Fig. 342), which is due to the damaging effect of the pressure on the corneal endothelium.

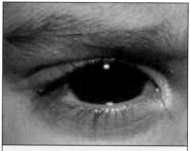

Fig. 343 Congenital glaucoma in an 8-month-old, with squinting, an enlarged globe, and subtle corneal edema causing an obscured view of the iris. Courtesy of Karen Joos, MD, PhD, Vanderbilt Eye Inst.

One type of juvenile glaucoma occurs in Sturge–Weber syndrome (Fig. 188), in which there is angiomatosis of the face and meninges with cerebral calcifications and seizures. The treatment of pediatric glaucoma is primarily surgical because medications are often ineffective and poorly tolerated in the long run.

Uvea

The uvea (Figs 344 and 345) is composed of the iris, ciliary body, and choroid. All three are contiguous, and pigmented with melanocytes.

The iris is a diaphragm that changes the size of the pupil by the action of the sympathetic dilator muscle and the cholinergic constrictor muscle.

Brushfield spots are normally occurring small, white-to-brown elevations on the peripheral

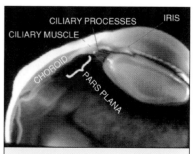

Fig. 344 Uvea. Courtesy of Stephen McCormick.

iris, more common in hazel or blue irises and in Down's syndrome (Fig. 346).

The ciliary body (Figs 345, 347, and 349) is made up of four clinically significant parts, as follows.

1 The anterior region serves as the site for insertion of the iris.
2 The ciliary processes secrete the aqueous (Figs 298 and 334) that nourishes the lens, cornea, and trabecular meshwork while maintaining intraocular pressure.
3 The smooth muscle changes the focus of the lens by contracting and decreasing tension on the zonules (Fig. 348).
4 The flat avascular pars plana serves as the best location to surgically enter the eye for intravitreal injections and vitreoretinal surgery (Figs 494, 495, 541, and 542).

The choroid has the highest blood flow and least oxygen extraction of any tissue in the body. Its purpose is to nourish the retina, which has one of the highest metabolic rates of any tissue in the body. Unlike the tree-like branching of the retinal vessels, the choroidal circulation appears to criss-cross in a tigroid-like appearance (Fig. 349). It is most easily visualized in advanced dry age-related macular degeneration (also called geographic AMD) after the retinal pigment layer disappears (Fig. 486) or in albinism where the retinal pigment never fully developed (Fig. 507).

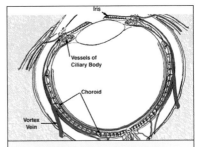

Fig. 345 The uvea is made up of the iris, ciliary body, and choroid. Courtesy of Pfizer Pharmaceuticals.

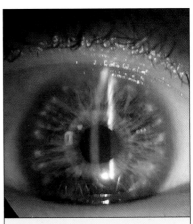

Fig. 346 Brushfield spots. Courtesy of University of Iowa, Eyerounds.org.

Malignant melanoma

A melanocyte tumor is the most common primary intraocular malignancy. It is unilateral and

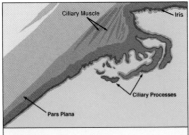

Fig. 347 Ciliary body. Courtesy of Pfizer Pharmaceuticals.

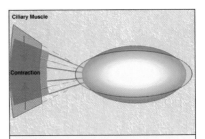

Fig. 348 Ciliary muscle focusing lens. Courtesy of Pfizer Pharmaceuticals.

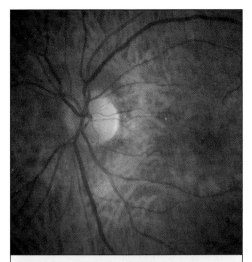

Fig. 349 Tigroid fundus with clearly visible, lightly pigmented choroidal vasculature. Courtesy of Elliot Davidoff, MD.

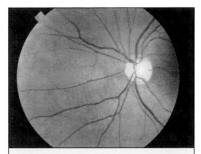

Fig. 350 Flat benign choroidal nevus.

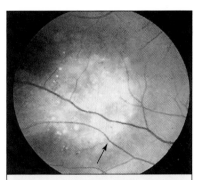

Fig. 351 Elevated malignant choroidal melanoma. Note change in direction as artery rises over tumor (↑).

develops from the choroid in 85% of cases, the ciliary body in 9%, and the iris in 6%. Unlike a benign nevus, which is usually a more uniform grey color and flat (Fig. 350), choroidal tumors are elevated and usually slate grey, but may be white to black with yellow-gold and uneven pigmentation (Fig. 351),. This must be distinguished from metastatic carcinoma to the eye, which is also most common in the choroid, but is usually lighter in color. The primary site is most often the breast or lung. Small intraocular malignancies are usually treated with a radioactive plaque (Fig. 352) which may preserve some vision. For larger tumors, the eye is sometimes removed enucleation (Figs 353, 354, and 394–397). If the tumor extends beyond the globe and is life threatening, an exenteration of the orbit is required. This rarely performed surgery is disfiguring and destructive. It could necessitate removal of the orbital contents, the eyelids, orbital walls, and periorbital structures (Fig. 355).

Patients with melanoma of the skin and elsewhere are often referred to eye physicians to rule out the eye as the primary site of origin of the tumor.

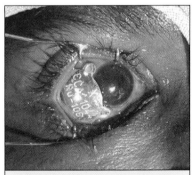

Fig. 352 Ruthenium radioactive plaque sewn or glued to the episclera of the eye is usually left in place for about 4 days and is used to treat smaller intraocular tumors. Courtesy of Dr Santosh G. Honor and Dr Surbhi Joshi, Prasad Eye Institute, Hyderabad, India.

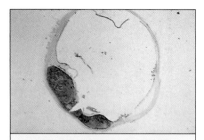

Fig. 353 Gross section of malignant melanoma treated with removal of the eye (enucleation).

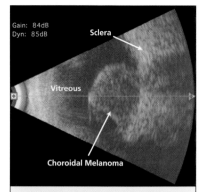

Fig. 354 B-scan ultrasound of a malignant choroidal melanoma showing typical dome-shaped growth which helps to confirm the diagnosis. The scan also shows its size and whether it extends beyond the sclera which will determine the type of treatment. This eye, with its massive tumor, was enucleated.

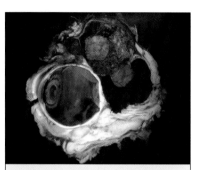

Fig. 355 Exenteration of the orbit for malignant melanoma extending beyond the sclera. *Source*: J.J. Ross et al., *Br. J. Ophthalmol.*, 2010, Vol. 94, No. 5.. Reproduced with permission of BMJ Publishing Group, Ltd.

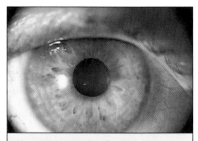

Fig. 356 Benign iris freckle.

Benign iris freckles (Fig. 356) and nevi are common, whereas malignant iris melanoma (Figs 357 and 358) is rare. Lesions become more suspicious if they are growing, elevated, vascularized, distorts the pupil, or cause inflammation, glaucoma, or cataracts.

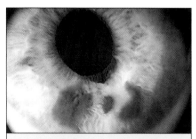

Fig. 357 Malignant iris melanoma with elevated lesions and distorted pupil.

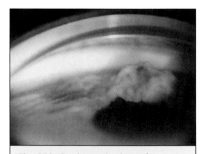

Fig. 358 Gonioscopic view of elevated iris melanoma. Courtesy of Michael P. Kelly.

Rubeosis iridis is a serious condition in which abnormal vessels grow on the surface of the iris (Figs 359 and 360) in response to ischemia associated with central retinal vein occlusion (or CRVO), proliferative diabetic retinopathy, or carotid artery occlusive disease. Untreated, the neovascularization could cause end stage glaucoma, painful enough to require multiple glaucoma surgeries or even removal of the eye (enucleation). Laser photocoagulation to destroy large areas of the retina may reduce ocular oxygen demand and cause regression of iris vessels.

An iris coloboma (Fig. 361) is due to failure of embryonic tissue to fuse inferiorly. It may also involve the choroid, lens, and optic nerve.

Inflammation of the uvea (uveitis)

Inflammations of the uvea are categorized by location: A, anterior (iritis); B, intermediate (ciliary body cyclitis); C, posterior (choroiditis); and D, panuveitis, involving all uveal structures. In 50% of cases, no cause is found. Most are treated with steroids and, less often, NSAIDs. Macular edema is the most common cause for loss of vision, but cataracts and glaucoma are also common.

Category A, iritis, inflammation of the iris, accounts for 92% of cases of uveitis. It causes pain, tearing, and photophobia. Signs include miosis (small pupil), perilimbal conjunctival injection (Figs 362, 363, and 367), and anterior chamber flare and cells (Fig. 363). Flare refers to the beam's milky appearance due to elevated protein. With the slit lamp on high magnification and a short, bright beam shone across the dark pupil, inflammatory cells are graded from trace to very many (4+).

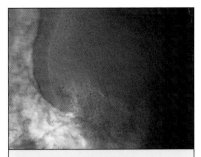

Fig. 359 Rubeosis iridis with neovascularization.

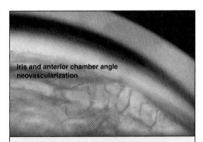

Fig. 360 Rubeosis iridis. These abnormal iris blood vessels scar the angle of the eye. They most often result from ischemic retinal diseases such as proliferative diabetic retinopathy and central retinal artery or vein occlusion.

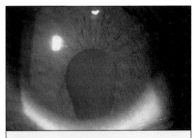

Fig. 361 Iris coloboma.

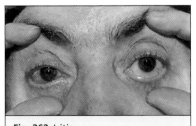

Fig. 362 Iritis.

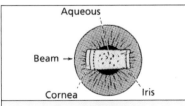

Fig. 363 Slit-beam view of flare and cells in anterior chamber.

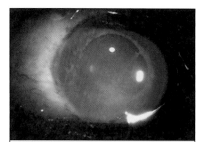

Fig. 364 Keratitic precipitates and posterior synechiae.

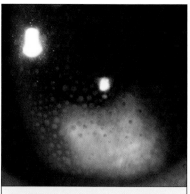

Fig. 365 Larger greasy yellowish keratitic precipitates called mutton-fat occur in sarcoidosis. Courtesy of University of Iowa, Eyerounds.org.

Deposits of inflammatory cells and protein on the corneal endothelium (Figs 364, 365, 367, and 370) are called keratitic precipitates (or KPs) and are often a sign that is present for more than a few days. Iritis usually reduces eye pressure due to depressed secretion of aqueous and increased uveoscleral outflow. Alternatively, eye pressure may become elevated if cellular debris obstructs the trabecular meshwork, or from the steroid used to treat the uveitis.

Another complication of iritis is posterior synechiae. These are adhesions between the iris and the lens capsule (Fig. 364). To prevent this, steroids, such as topical prednisolone 1% (Pred Forte), are given to prevent a fibrinous sticky aqueous. Medrysone (HMS 1%), fluorometholone 0.25% (FML Forte), and loteprednol 0.5% (Lotimax) are three examples of steroids with less pressure-elevating effects, but are less potent. Frequency and strength of medication depends on the severity of the condition.

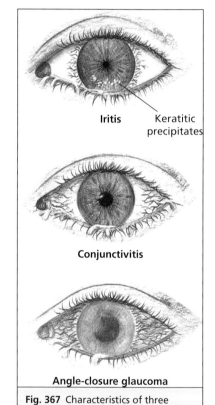

Iritis   Keratitic precipitates

Conjunctivitis

Angle-closure glaucoma

Fig. 367 Characteristics of three causes of an inflamed eye (see table, opposite).

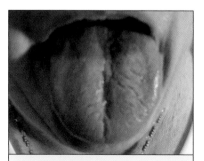

Fig. 366 Patient with Behcet's disease with ulcers and fissures on her tongue. She complained of constant burning in mouth.

Common causes of an injected conjunctiva			
	Iritis	*Conjunctivitis*	*Acute glaucoma*
Symptom	Pain, photophobia	Gritty, itching	Pain (often severe), photophobia
Discharge	Tearing	Pus, mucus, or tears	Tearing
Pupil	Miotic	Normal	Mid-dilated
Injection	Limbal	Diffuse	Diffuse and limbal
Cornea	Keratitic precipitates	Clear	Steamy cornea
Pressure	Usually low	Normal	Elevated
Anterior chamber	Flare and cells	Normal	Shallow

Anti-inflammatories

Corticosteroids have been the mainstay of therapy for ocular inflammation since their initial use in the 1950s. They are commonly used to treat uveitis, post-operative inflammation, allergic and infectious conjunctivitis, keratitis, scleritis, episcleritis, and Grave's orbitopathy. They are commonly given by eye drop to treat anterior uveitis. Periocular steroid injections – subconjunctival or retrobulbar – are used for severe anterior uveitis, intermediate uveitis, and posterior uveitis. The drug passes easily through the sclera, bypassing the corneal and conjunctival barriers. Chronic, more severe, posterior uveitis may be treated with an intravitreal steroid implant, especially if it is chronic and causing macular edema. Oral steroids may also be tried in resistant cases. Systemic immune-suppressive drugs – most commonly methotrexate – are sometimes substituted for oral steroids, since they are safer for long-term use.

Local side effects of corticosteroids include cataracts, glaucoma, and activation of herpes keratitis. Systemic side effects include reduced immunity, osteoporosis, and exacerbation of diabetes or gastric ulcers. Topical NSAID drops, such as generic ketorolac 0.5%, are less effective and may be used in addition to the steroid or as a stand-alone treatment, especially in glaucoma patients, since they don't elevate eye pressure.

Cycloplegics, such as cyclopentolate 1% or longer-acting atropine 1%, are instilled to keep the pupil dilated thereby minimizing the chance of posterior synechiae and also to relieve pain and photophobia due to ciliary muscle spasm.

Anticholinergics

Anticholinergic	Action time	Primary use
Atropine 0.5–1%	±2 weeks	Prolonged or severe anterior uveitis
Scopolamine 0.25% (hyoscine 0.25%)	±4 days	Alternative when allergic to atropine
Homatropine 2–5%	±2 days	Anterior uveitis
Cyclopentolate (Cyclogyl) 1–2%	±1 day	Cycloplegic retinoscopy; rapid onset (30 minutes)
Tropicamide (Mydriacyl) 0.5%	±6 hours	Often used with phenylephrine 2.5% or 10% for pupil dilation

Iritis is caused most often by intraocular surgery, blunt ocular trauma, and corneal ulcers, abrasions, and foreign bodies. Human leukocyte antigen (HLA-B27) is found in 2–9% of normal persons. Of this small group of individuals possessing the HLA-B27 antigen, 20% are predisposed to autoimmune disorders. Iritis may be associated with the following five HLA-B27-positive autoimmune diseases:

1 ankylosing spondylitis (mostly males with arthritis of the lower spine, of whom 95% are HLA-B27-positive),
2 juvenile idiopathic arthritis,
3 reactive arthritis (formerly Reiter's syndrome), in males with urethritis and conjunctivitis,
4 inflammatory bowel disease,
5 psoriatic arthritis.

Causes that are not related to HLA-B27 levels are toxoplasmosis, sarcoidosis, Lyme disease, influenza, lymphoma, AIDS, herpes simplex and zoster (shingles), and Behcet's disease (ulcers in the mouth [Fig. 366] and genitals). There are other even rarer etiologies. Therefore, careful clinical judgment is needed in determining the timing and extent of the workup, taking into consideration cost, severity, chronicity, and associated medical history (see table, p. 126, A workup for uveitis, for a basic workup).

Patients with juvenile idiopathic arthritis and chronic iritis often develop a band of calcification in Bowman's membrane known as band keratopathy (Fig. 368). It also occurs in sarcoidosis and hypervitaminosis D. It may be removed

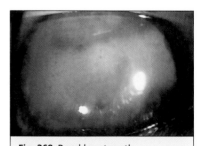

Fig. 368 Band keratopathy.

by using a technique called chelation in which the calcium is dissolved by applying ethylenediaminetetraacetic acid (EDTA) to the cornea.

Category B for inflammations of the uvea, inflammation of the ciliary body (cyclitis), is also called intermediate uveitis, and is characterized 80% of the time by having cells in the vitreous. It causes pain and decreased eye pressure. Cells in the vitreous reduce vision. It may be infectious, inflammatory, or neoplastic. Multiple sclerosis, sarcoidosis (Figs 369–378), cigarette smoking, trauma, Lyme disease, and syphilis should be considered; however, idiopathic pars planitis is common.

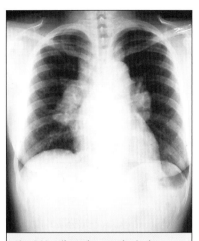

Fig. 369 Hilar adenopathy is the number one sign of sarcoidosis occurring in 75% of cases. Courtesy of Aman K. Farr, MD, and *Arch. Ophthalmol.*, May 2000, Vol. 118, Nos 1–6, p. 729. Copyright 2000, American Medical Association. All rights reserved.

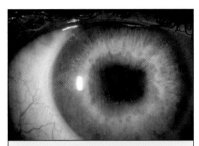

Fig. 370 Iritis occurs in 25% of patients with sarcoidosis and is the number one ocular finding. Above are large smooth (mutton-fat) keratitic precipitates and an irregular pupil due to posterior synechiae. Courtesy of Rhonda Curtis, CRA, COT, Washington University Medical School, St. Louis, MO.

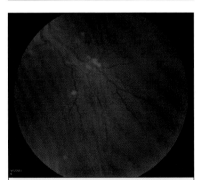

Fig. 371 Sarcoidosis with intermediate uveitis and "snowballs" of inflammatory cells in the peripheral vitreous. Courtesy of Julia Monsonego, CRA, Wills Eye Hospital.

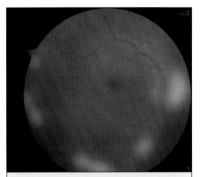

Fig. 372 Intermediate uveitis (pars planitis) with snowballing of inflammatory cells on the pars plana. Courtesy of Careen Lowder, MD, Cole Eye Institute.

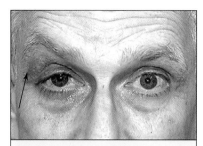

Fig. 373 CT scan of sarcoidosis with bilaterally enlarged lacrimal glands (↑). This patient also had lung, skin, conjunctiva, and kidney involvement.

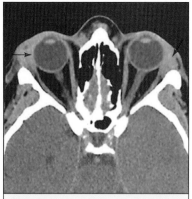

Fig. 374 Visibly enlarged right lacrimal gland (↑). Notice elevated right brow and ptosis.

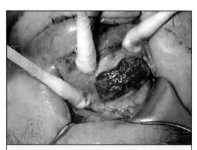

Fig. 375 A lacrimal gland biopsy often helps confirm the diagnosis of sarcoidosis.

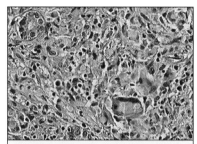

Fig. 376 Light photomicrograph of lacrimal gland infiltrated with non-caseating granuloma.

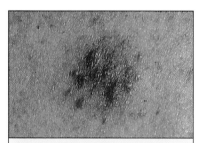

Fig. 377 Tender erythematous subcutaneous sarcoid nodule (Figs 373–376). Courtesy of Dr John Woogend and *Arch. Ophthalmol.*, May 2007, Vol. 125, pp. 707–709. Copyright 2007, American Medical Association. All rights reserved.

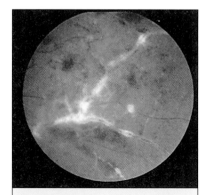

Fig. 378 Sarcoidosis with vasculitis causing "candle-wax" drippings on vessel. Courtesy of Joseph Walsh, MD.

Sarcoidosis

Sarcoidosis is a systemic disease of unknown etiology characterized in 75% of patients by granulomatous inflammation of the lung (Fig. 369). It also affects skin (Fig. 377), peripheral nerves, liver, kidney, and other tissues. The main ocular finding is iritis often associated with large, greasy (mutton-fat) keratitic precipitates (Figs 365 and 370). Lacrimal gland granulomas (Figs 373–376), intermediate uveitis, and vasculitis (Fig. 378) occur less frequently. It is usually treated with local or systemic corticosteroids.

Category C for inflammations of the uvea, choroiditis, is characterized by white exudates extending onto the retina. It is sometimes obscured from view by cells in the vitreous. It leads to chorioretinal atrophy with pigment mottling (Fig. 379). Often no cause is found, but the following etiologies should be considered.

Causes of choroiditis

1 Bacterial: syphilis (Figs 382–386) tuberculosis.
2 Viral: herpes simplex, cytomegalovirus in 25% of AIDS patients (Figs 389 and 390).
3 Fungal: histoplasmosis (Fig. 380), candidiasis.
4 Parasitic: *Toxoplasma*, *Toxocara* (Fig. 379).
5 Immunosuppression: AIDS predisposes to several of the above.
6 Behcet's disease (mouth and genital ulcers with dermatitis) (Fig. 366); sympathetic ophthalmia (see Fig. 124).

Choroiditis often requires subconjunctival intravitreal or systemic steroids, especially when it threatens the macula, optic nerve, or the associated vitritis is a potential source of membrane formation.

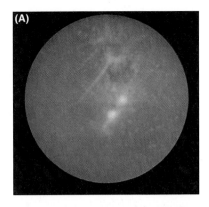

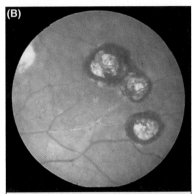

Fig. 379 (A) *Toxoplasma gondii* chorioretinitis often reactivates next to old lesion. One quarter of the US population is seropositive for toxoplasmosis, but only 2% of these will develop eye disease. Up to 25% of lamb and pork in the USA has been reported to harbor cysts. Infection is spread by congenital or oral transmission. Active lesion appears as a "headlight in the fog." (B) Old toxoplasmosis scar: sclera visible through atrophic retina and choroid.

Nematodes

Parasitic worms, sometimes referred to as microfilaria, may infect humans (Fig. 381). *Toxocara canis* and *Toxocara cati* are microfilaria transmitted by the oral ingestion of ova. Toddlers may ingest them by playing on the

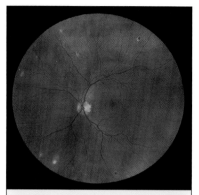

Fig. 380 Histoplasmosis with multiple punched out chorioretinitic lesions called "histospots." Courtesy of Alexis Smith, CRT, OCT-T, Kellogg Eye Center, Michigan.

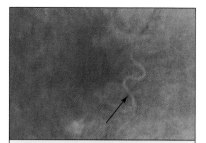

Fig. 381 Unknown southeastern US subretinal nematode (↑) causing neuroretinitis. Courtesy of J. Donald M. Gass, MD, and *Arch. Ophthalmol.*, Nov. 1983, Vol. 101(3), pp. 1689–1697. Copyright 1983, American Medical Association. All rights reserved.

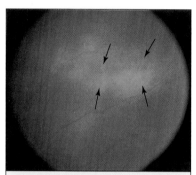

Fig. 382 Syphilitic, yellow, flat chorioretinal lesions. Courtesy of Thomas R. Friberg, MD, and *Arch. Ophthalmol.*, Nov. 1989, Vol. 107, pp. 1571–1572. Copyright 1989, American Medical Association. All rights reserved.

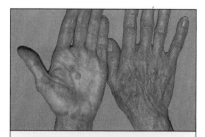

Fig. 383 Maculopapular syphilitic eruption involving palms.

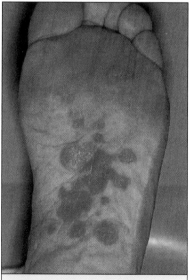

Fig. 384 Maculopapular syphilitic eruption involving soles.

ground where animals have defecated and adults may ingest them by eating unwashed vegetables.

Don't confuse the *Toxocara* nematode, which is an extracellular parasite, with the other similar-sounding parasite, *Toxoplasma*, which lives inside the cell. However, what toxocariasis and toxoplasmosis have in common is that both may cause severe intraocular inflammation.

Onchocerca volvulus, found 95% of the time in Africa, afflicts people living along riverbanks. It is responsible for 270,000 cases of blindness caused by scarring of the cornea, optic neuritis, and chorioretinitis. The disease is often called "river blindness." Another African worm – *Loa loa* – can migrate to the lids and conjunctiva where it can live for up to 17 years and cause inflammation.

Syphilis

This infectious disease (Figs 382–386), caused by *Treponema pallidum*, is usually transmitted through sexual contact. It can infect any organ of the body. Ocular involvement usually includes the uvea, resulting in iritis, cyclitis, and chorioretinitis. Neurosyphilis could involve all the cranial nerves and cause the pupillary response called the Argyll Robertson pupil. Here, the pupils may be irregularly constricted with decreased or absent response to light, but a normal near reflex. The pupil dilates poorly with mydriatics.

Sadly, the incidence of syphilis increased almost every year between 2000 and 2014 in males having sex with other males.

Human immunodeficiency virus (HIV)

This retrovirus invades and inactivates the CD4+ T-lymphocytes of the immune system. Initially, it may cause weight loss, headache, malaise, fever, chills, and lymphadenopathy. When the CD4+ T-cells drop from the normal of 500–1500 cells/mm^3 to less than 200 cells/mm^3, the acquired immune deficiency syndrome (AIDS) begins. AIDS occurs in 38.3% of those infected with HIV within a year of diagnosis and 45% within 3 years. Up to 90% of adults in the USA harbor herpes simplex virus, 40–80% have cytomegalovirus (CMV) (Fig. 390), and 25% have antibodies to *Toxoplasma gondii*. These three opportunistic organisms are among the most common to become virulent in immune-comprised patients with AIDS.

If the CD4+ T-cell count is >200 cells/mm^3 with no ocular disease, a yearly eye exam

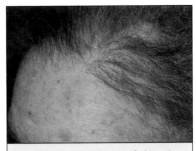

Fig. 385 Syphilitic zones of alopecia prompted patient to wear a wig.

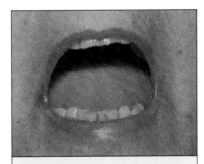

Fig. 386 Syphilitic painless mucous membrane ulcers occurred at the corners of patient's mouth.

is adequate; otherwise, the patient is at increased risk from opportunistic infection and should be examined every 4 months. Highly active antiretroviral therapy (HAART) should be started at the detection of HIV virus. Without treatment, nearly every patient with HIV will get AIDS. Medications or the disease could cause uveitis, vitritis, epiretinal membranes, or acute retinal necrosis that could lead to retinal detachment. HAART therapy, together with Vitrasert (ganciclovir) intravitreal implants, have resulted in a reduction in both HIV- and CMV-associated mortality and a 90% reduction in retinitis complications in the USA. Kaposi's sarcoma (Figs 387 and 388) is the malignancy seen most often in AIDS. There is a non-tender purple nodule on the skin or conjunctiva. Rx: radiation or excision.

Sympathetic ophthalmia

This is a rare condition. It refers to a traumatic or surgical injury to the uvea of one eye resulting in a chronic, immune panuveitis involving both eyes. A penetrating injury through the corneoscleral wall is referred to as an open-globe injury (Figs 391–393). Handle the eye with minimal probing. Place the patient at rest with bilateral shields that exert no pressure and start intravenous broad-spectrum antibiotics. Call the eye surgeon immediately. If the uvea or retina are extruded from the eye and it cannot be repaired, the eye is removed (enucleated) (Fig. 394). A spherical prosthesis is then placed in the orbit and covered with conjunctiva (Figs 395–397). A removable scleral prosthesis fit by an ocularist is painted to match the other eye and is placed on the conjunctiva. Enucleation should be performed within 10 days of the injury to prevent sympathetic ophthalmia. If the rare occurrence of sympathetic ophthalmia does occur, corticosteroids and immunomodulatory therapy may be required for many years and possibly decades.

A blind, severely atrophic anatomically disfigured eye called phthisis bulbi may be removed for cosmetic reasons or to relieve pain.

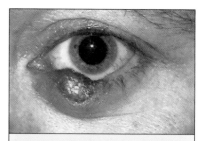

Fig. 387 Kaposi's sarcoma of skin in AIDS due to the opportunistic infection by herpesvirus 8. Courtesy of Jerry Shields, MD.

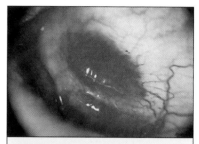

Fig. 388 Kaposi's sarcoma of conjunctiva. Courtesy of Jerry Shields, MD.

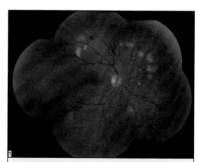

Fig. 389 AIDS retinopathy with cotton-wool spots and intraretinal hemorrhages occurs in 50% of patients with AIDS. There is no treatment. Courtesy of Julia Monsonego, CRA Wills Eye Hospital.

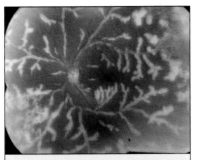

Fig. 390 Cytomegalovirus (CMV) is the most frequent opportunistic infection in patients with AIDS. Retinitis is a significant risk factor for mortality. This case shows frosted retinal angitis. Courtesy of Harry Flynn, MD, and *Retinal Physician*, Oct. 2010, Vol. 7, No. 8, p. 67.

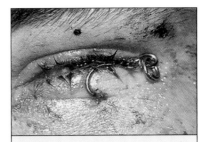

Fig. 391 Fish hook in eye.

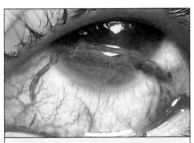

Fig. 392 Open-globe injury through corneoscleral wall with prolapse of iris and ciliary body.

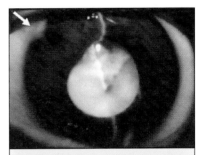

Fig. 393 Penetrating injury through iris and lens capsule with secondary cataract.

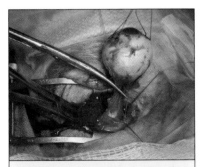

Fig. 394 Enucleation: the eye is removed by first exposing and then severing the insertions of the six extraocular muscles. Then the optic nerve is cut as shown above. An eye may be removed when it is blind, painful, cosmetically unappealing, or harbors a tumor. Courtesy of Jeffrey Nerad, MD.

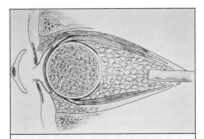

Fig. 395 Silicone orbital implant with scleral prosthesis. Courtesy of Integrated Orbital Implants, Inc.

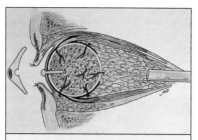

Fig. 396 Porous hydroxyapatite implant allows ingrowth of blood vessels to prevent migration or extrusion. Muscles may be sutured to implant to provide more normal movement. Courtesy of Integrated Orbital Implants, Inc.

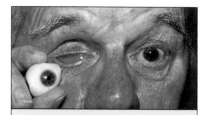

Fig. 397 Enucleated socket with scleral prosthesis.

A workup for uveitis

A workup for uveitis is necessary when there is no obvious cause and if it is prolonged or severe. The following screening tests for most common causes should be considered depending on the geographic location, age of patient, and other signs and symptoms. The patient should also be referred to a primary care physician suggesting reasons for this workup with your recommendations.

Diagnosis	Major clues	Laboratory evaluation
AIDS	Malaise, weight loss, lymphadenopathy, and signs of infection, especially toxoplasmosis, cytomegalovirus, and herpes simplex	HIV-1, HIV-2, antibody screen
Ankylosing spondylitis	Often males with lower back pain	HLA-B27, sacroiliac and lumbar spinal x-ray
Anterior uveitis (HLA-B27+)	Associated with ankylosing spondylitis, inflammatory bowel disease, psoriasis, reactive arthritis (formerly Reiter's syndrome), juvenile idiopathic arthritis	HLA-B27
Behcet's disease	Young adults with mouth and genital ulcers, and skin lesions	HLA-B51
Coccidioidomycosis	Chorioretinitis, fever, cough; endemic along coast of California, Mexico, and South America	Serum antibodies
Cytomegalovirus	Most commonly in AIDS; severe retinitis	CMV antibody titer
Histoplasmosis (fungus)	Multiple, small, chorioretinal lesions (histo spots) (Fig. 380) linked to bird droppings along the Ohio and Mississippi river valleys	Histoplasmin skin test
Juvenile idiopathic arthritis	Children, fever with hepatosplenomegaly (Still's disease)	+ANA 75% of time

Continued on p. 127

Diagnosis	Major clues	Laboratory evaluation
Lyme disease	Tick bite, skin rash, arthropathy, neurologic symptoms, mostly in New England and mid-Atlantic states	Serum anti-*Borrelia burgdorferi* antibodies
Lymphoma	Vitritis and anterior uveitis	MRI, lumbar puncture, and/or vitreous cytology
Multiple sclerosis	Intermediate uveitis, neurologic symptoms, especially optic neuritis	MRI of brain
Polyarteritis nodosa	Systemic necrotizing vasculitis causing fatigue, myalgia, weight loss, nephritis, fever, arthralgia, iritis, keratitis, scleritis	↑ ESR, biopsy of artery confirms diagnosis, ↑ blood urea nitrogen
Reactive arthritis (formerly Reiter's syndrome)	Iridocyclitis, urethritis, arthritis	75% (+) HLA-B27, elevated ESR, ANA
Rheumatoid arthritis	Joint pain, anemia	Rheumatoid factor +85% of time (elevated ESR)
Sarcoidosis	Breathing disorder most common, panuveitis, lymph node enlargement	Chest x-ray, biopsy of skin, conjunctiva, lymph node, or lacrimal gland; serum ACE
Sjögren's syndrome	Mainly women, dry eye and mouth, arthritis	Anti-SSA/Ro and anti-SSB, subtypes of ANA
Syphilis	Retinitis, choroiditis, multitude of systemic symptoms	RPR or VDRL
Systemic lupus erythematosus	90% women, macular rash, oral and nasal ulcers, discoid lupus, arthritis, pleurisy, pericarditis	ANA is + in 95% of SLE
Toxoplasmosis (intracellular protozoa)	Very common; anterior and posterior uveitis; often in AIDS	Serum anti-*Toxoplasma gondii* antibodies: 23% of US have + antibody
Toxocariasis (roundworm)	Posterior uveitis in toddlers with exposure to dog or cat	6% of US positive for serum ELISA antibodies to *Toxocara*; eosinophilia
Tuberculosis (infects 20–43% of world population)	Cough, fever, weight loss, malaise, and sweats	Chest x-ray, PPD skin test
Wegner's granulomatosis (now called granulomatosis with polyangiitis, GPA)	Uveitis and retinitis; often involves upper and lower respiratory tracts, but also kidneys and CNS; orbital pseudotumor (p. 74) occurs in 45% of patients	Chest x-ray shows cavitary lesions and pneumonitis; biopsy any involved tissue, anti-neutrophil cytoplasmic antibody positive in only 40%

ACE, angiotensin converting enzyme; ANA, antinuclear antibody; anti-SSA, SSB, types A and B anti-Sjögren's syndrome antinuclear antibodies; ESR, erythyrocyte sedimentation rate; PPD, purified protein derivative skin test; RPR, rapid plasma reagin; VDRL, Venereal Disease Research Laboratory.

Cataracts

A cataract is a cloudy lens. It should be suspected when the patient complains of blurry vision and there is a hazy view of the retina with an ophthalmoscope. The lens consists of an outside capsule surrounding a soft cortical substance and a hard inner nucleus (Fig. 398). The diagnosis is confirmed with a slit lamp and described in the following ways.

1 By etiology: it is usually due to aging, but may be congenital or brought on by radiation, ultraviolet light, diabetes, trauma (perforation of capsule) (see Fig. 393), or steroids. Steroid used to treat chronic iritis in juvenile idiopathic arthritis almost always causes cataracts. There is twice the incidence in cigarette smokers. Juvenile cataracts are rare. Fifty eight percent are idiopathic, 13% are traumatic, and 12% are inherited, most commonly with Down's syndrome. There are over 100 congenital syndromes associated with cataracts. All children should have a full eye exam before age 4–5 to uncover cataracts, and, more commonly, amblyopia. Children with rare syndromes should be checked even earlier if there are any unusual systemic signs and symptoms.

2 By location in lens: cortex (Fig. 399), nucleus, or posterior subcapsule (often due to steroids; Fig. 400).

3 By color or pattern: the infantile inherited type is located in or around the nucleus, and is often non-progressive (Fig. 401). A mature, dark brown lens is often hard and difficult to break up (Fig. 402) during cataract surgery.

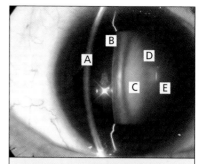

Fig. 398 Slit lamp view of lens: A, cornea; B, anterior capsule; C, nucleus; D, posterior cortex; E, posterior capsule. Courtesy of Takashi Fujkado, MD.

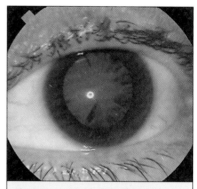

Fig. 399 Anterior cortical spokes.

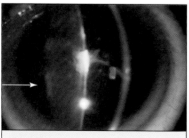

Fig. 400 Posterior subcapsular cataract.

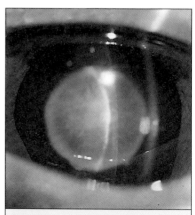

Fig. 401 Congenital (zonular) cataract surrounded by clear cortex.

A cataract raises two questions. Is it responsible for the decreased vision? Is it ripe? Ripe is the layperson's term for whether surgery is indicated. In most cases, a surgeon waits for a reduction in vision to 20/50 or worse, but indications vary with the patient's needs. Surgery is usually elective except in the rare cases of a mature lens that might rupture or is already leaking (Fig. 403), or with a dislocated lens in imminent danger of dropping into the vitreous or anterior chamber. Lens dislocation (Fig. 404) is due to rupture of the zonules. It occurs with trauma or may be associated with Marfan's disease, homocystinuria, or syphilis. Cataract surgery is performed as an outpatient procedure using local anesthesia, and is the number one major surgery performed in the USA in the elderly. The cornea is entered with a blade or laser, making a three-plane incision to minimize chance of leakage and the need for sutures (Fig. 405). When wound closure is not adequate, sutures or ReSure, a hydrogel sealant, may be used. The latter lasts 2–3 days.

The anterior lens capsule is then removed (Figs 406 and 408). The majority of the time a continuous tear capsulotomy, called capsulorrhexis, is used. However, the femtosecond laser is possibly more precise for performing this step. The hard nucleus is rarely extracted in one piece (Fig. 407). To facilitate removal of the nucleus through a small wound, it is manually fragmented (Fig. 410) or liquified with a phacoemulsifier, which has a tip that vibrates 40,000 times per second (Fig. 409) (phaco- is a prefix referring to the lens). Phacoemulsification's disadvantage is that it requires a lot of energy to liquefy a hard nucleus. This could damage the corneal endothelium or the delicate posterior lens capsule.

A less expensive alternative to phacoemulsification that is more commonly used in the developing world is manual fracture of the nucleus. A platform is placed under the hard nucleus and a chopper is placed on top. Pushing down divides the nucleus (Figs 410 and 411) into two pieces, so it can be removed through a smaller incision.

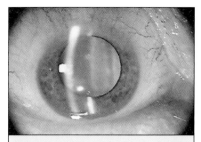

Fig. 402 Brunescent (brown) cataract.

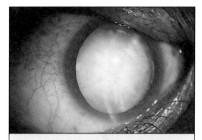

Fig. 403 Mature lens dislocated into the anterior chamber, obscuring pupil and iris.

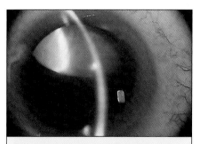

Fig. 404 Superiorly dislocated lens.

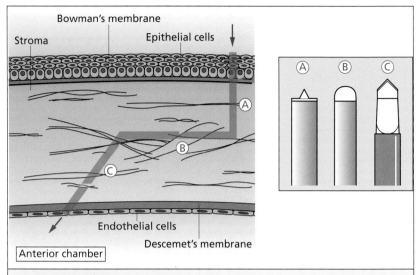

Fig. 405 A three-plane corneal incision for entering the eye during cataract surgery. Blade A is guarded to create a uniform mid-depth incision approximately 3–6 mm in length. Blade B is crescent shaped for a 4 mm dissection of corneal lamellae. A downward motion with the keratome (blade C) enters the anterior chamber.

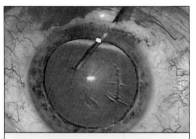

Fig. 406 Anterior capsulotomy: 50 punctures of anterior capsule prior to removal. Courtesy of Richard Tipperman, MD, and Stephen Lichtenstein, MD.

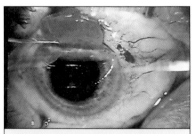

Fig. 407 Removal of hard nucleus in one piece. Courtesy of Richard Tipperman, MD, and Stephen Lichtenstein, MD.

After the nucleus is removed by either method, the soft cortex is aspirated (Fig. 412) and the eye is referred to as aphakic. A spectacle lens of about +12.0 D would be required to focus the eye, but it is thick and magnifies the image 33% larger than the normal eye, so that the two eyes cannot fuse. A contact lens that magnifies the image to a lesser degree than a spectacle

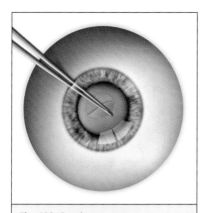

Fig. 408 Continuous tear capsulotomy (capsulorrhexis).

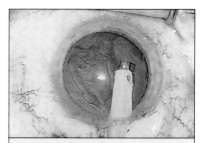

Fig. 409 Removal of nucleus by phacoemulsification. Courtesy of Richard Tipperman, MD, and Stephen Lichtenstein, MD.

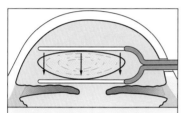

Fig. 410 Manual phacofragmentation of nucleus after dislocation into anterior chamber.

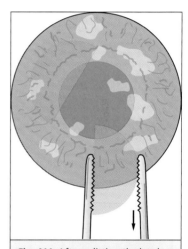

Fig. 411 After splitting the hard nucleus, it is removed in two pieces with toothed forceps. Note the white cortex still to be aspirated.

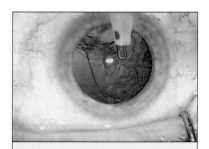

Fig. 412 After removing the nucleus by either technique, the surrounding cortex is removed with irrigation and aspiration. Courtesy of Richard Tipperman, MD, and Stephen Lichtenstein, MD.

lens can minimize the problem of image size disparity (aniseikonia) and allow binocular vision. However, contact lenses are impractical with elderly patients. Therefore, an acrylic or silicone lens implant of about +18.0 D is inserted into the eye to restore distance vision and the eye is then referred to as pseudophakic. A-scan ultrasound is used to measure the anteroposterior diameter of the eye. This length, together with the corneal curvature, as determined with a keratometer, gives the exact power of the intraocular lens implant needed. Intraocular lens use is presently being evaluated as to its safety profile in infants as young as 7 months of age, but has gained wide acceptance after 2 years of age and is commonplace after age 7.

The lens is usually placed behind the iris (Figs 413–415), unless the posterior capsule or zonules are torn and can't support it. In these cases, it is placed in front of the iris (Fig. 416). This eye is now in focus for distance, but requires a spectacle for focus at near.

Multifocal lens implants that focus the eye for near and far are expensive, can cause glare, and are only used in about 8% of selected patients so that they might be spectacle-free. One type has alternating rings with different refractive powers (Fig. 418) and the other changes its refractive power by shifting its position with accommodative stimulation

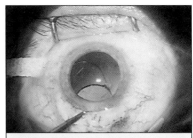

Fig. 413 Insertion of rigid lens through 6 mm incision. Courtesy of Richard Tipperman, MD, and Stephen Lichtenstein, MD.

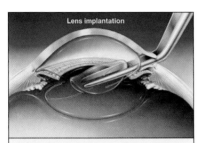

Fig. 414 Foldable implant inserted through 3.2 mm incision is overwhelmingly preferred.

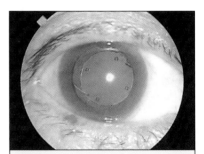

Fig. 415 Posterior chamber lens behind iris and in the capsular bag is first choice.

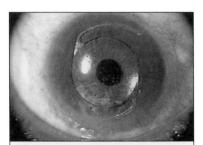

Fig. 416 Anterior chamber lens, sometimes used when the posterior capsule of zonules are damaged during surgery and can't support air in the capsule (bag) implant.

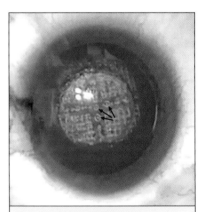

Fig. 417 Femtosecond laser-assisted grid fragmentation allows surgeons to soften the nucleus so that phacoemulsification requires less damaging ultrasound power. Courtesy of Richard Witlin, MD.

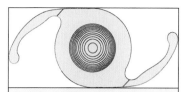

Fig. 418 ReSTOR multifocal intraocular lens with 12 concentric steps of focusing power, which allows focus from far to near. It could cause halos and glare, especially at night.

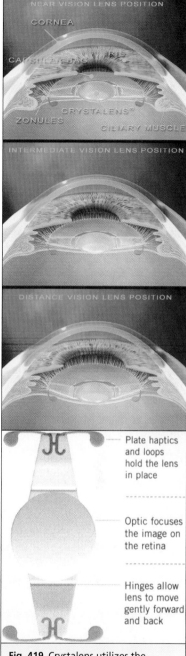

Plate haptics and loops hold the lens in place

Optic focuses the image on the retina

Hinges allow lens to move gently forward and back

Fig. 419 Crystalens utilizes the natural action of the ciliary muscle during accommodation to move the optic of the implanted lens forward to focus for near.

to the ciliary body muscle (Fig. 419). In eyes with significant amounts of astigmatism, a more expensive toric implant may be inserted (Fig. 420). Care must be taken in aligning the axis and preventing post-operative rotation.

Laser-assisted cataract surgery

In 2014, 5% of cataracts were performed using laser. The increased cost and additional time has made the routine use of femtosecond-laser-assisted cataract extraction quite controversial. Advocates cite four advantages.

1 The laser facilitates capsulotomy (capsulorrhexis). Manually performed "can opener" (Fig. 406) or continuous circular tear (Fig. 408) capsulotomy are difficult to perform and are not as precise as the laser in reproducing the size and centration of the opening.
2 Emulsification of a hard nucleus with conventional phacofragmentation alone requires extra ultrasound energy. By presoftening and segmenting the nucleus with a laser (Fig. 417) less energy is needed thus protecting intraocular structures, especially the corneal endothelium. The fragments created are of a more predictable size. making aspiration into the phaco tip more predictable.
3 Astigmatism of up to 1.50 D can be corrected during cataract surgery (with a blade), creating one or two partial-thickness arcuate corneal limbus-relaxing incisions (Fig. 72) of about 2–3 clock hours. The laser is thought by some to be more precise than a blade.

4 Most cataract surgeries are performed by entering the eye through a clear peripheral corneal incision of about 3 mm in length. Initial reports indicate that the laser-cut incision may be less prone to wound leaking, although this is debatable.

Some complications of cataract surgery

1 The posterior capsule may opacify months to years after cataract extraction in 30% of cases and is called a secondary cataract (Fig. 421). It may be opened with a YAG laser (Fig. 422).

2 If the zonules tear, the implant could dislocate (Figs 423 and 424) in 0.3–3.0% of

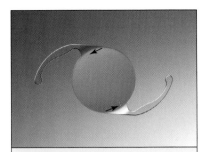

Fig. 420 AcrySof IQ Toric intraocular lens. A marker is first used to mark the axis of the astigmatism on the cornea of the eye. The lens is then inserted so the marks on the lens and eye line up. Image courtesy of Alcon Laboratories, Inc.

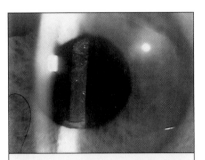

Fig. 421 Secondary cataract. Courtesy of Richard Tipperman, MD, and Stephen Lichtenstein, MD.

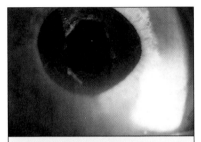

Fig. 422 YAG laser capsulotomy for secondary cataract of posterior capsule. Courtesy of Richard Tipperman, MD, and Stephen Lichtenstein, MD.

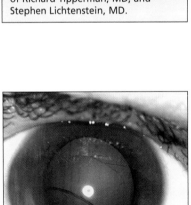

Fig. 423 Dislocated intraocular lens due to weakened zonules. Courtesy of Elliot Davidoff, MD.

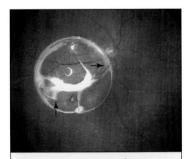

Fig. 424 Lens implant (↑ lens haptic) and capsular bag dislocated into the vitreous after traumatic tearing of the zonules. Courtesy of S. Parthasarethi, MD, and *Arch. Ophthalmol.*, Sept. 2007, Vol. 125, p. 1240. Copyright 2007, American Medical Association. All rights reserved.

cases. These implants have to supported with sutures to the iris or sclera or placed in front of the iris (Fig. 425).

3 The corneal endothelium could be damaged, resulting in corneal edema (Fig. 245). It is the most common reason for corneal endothelium transplant surgery, DSEK (Figs 252–256).

4 Retinal detachment (Figs 531 and 532) occurs in 1–2% of cataract surgeries.

5 Infectious endophthalmitis (Figs 426 and 427) is a serious, potentially blinding, complication of cataract surgery or any penetrating intraocular injury or injection. A culture is taken of the aqueous and vitreous and topical, subconjunctival, and intravitreal antibiotics are administered immediately. Fortunately, it only occurs in 1 in 1000 cataract surgeries.

6 Macular edema occurs in 2–60% of cataract surgeries, reducing vision during the post-operative period. It fortunately resolves in almost all cases (see Fig. 491).

A vitrectomy is often performed to obtain a sample for culture and to prevent formation of membranes that cause vitreoretinal traction, which could result in a retinal detachment.

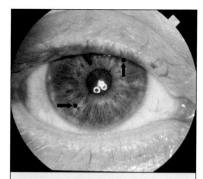

Fig. 425 Dislocated posterior chamber lens with haptics sutured to iris. Suturing to sclera is also common place and results in similar final outcomes, although the latter takes longer to perform.

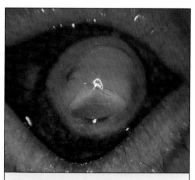

Fig. 427 Severe endophthalmitis with visibly dislocated lens implant in anterior chamber. Courtesy of Julia Monsonego, CRA, Wills Eye Hospital.

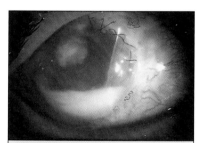

Fig. 426 Endophthalmitis with hypopyon following cataract surgery.

Chapter 7
The retina and vitreous

Retinal anatomy

The retina is the sensory layer of the eye, extending from the optic disk to the ora serrata (Figs 428–431).

Light stimulates 120 million rods, which are mainly located in the peripheral retina. They are very sensitive to small amounts of light critical for night vision. Five million cones, located primarily in the fovea and macula, are responsible for color vision and the acute vision needed to read. Both receptor types transmit the message to the ganglion cell on the retinal surface. The long ganglion cell axons exit the eye in the optic nerve, which synapses in the brain (Fig. 432).

The macula

The macula is rich in cones and is the most sensitive area of the retina. The retinal vessels terminate at its margin, and in its center is an avascular pit called the fovea, which produces a light reflex. This reflex decreases with age, and its absence in a young individual with a visual disturbance could indicate macular dysfunction. When the macula is destroyed, the vision is 20/200 at best.

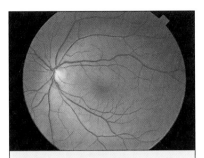

Fig. 428 Posterior retinal landmarks.

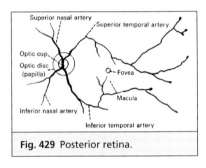

Fig. 429 Posterior retina.

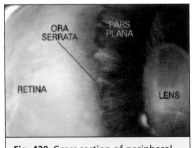

Fig. 430 Gross section of peripheral retina.

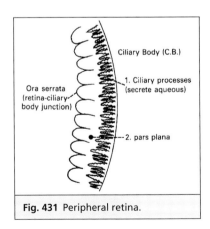

Fig. 431 Peripheral retina.

Manual for Eye Examination and Diagnosis, Ninth edition. Mark Leitman.

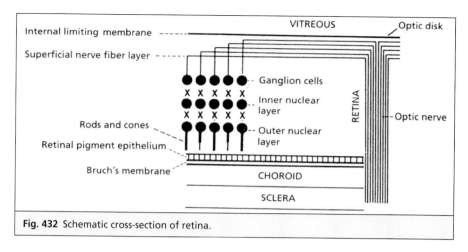

Fig. 432 Schematic cross-section of retina.

The optic disk

The optic disk is normally orange-red with a yellow cup at its center. The retinal artery and vein pass through the optic cup and bifurcate on the surface of the disk. Proliferation of the retinal pigment epithelium (RPE) at the disk margin is a normal finding (Fig. 433).

In axial myopia, the eye is increased in length and the retina may be dragged away from the optic disk margin, exposing the sclera. This is called a myopic conus or crescent (Fig. 434). In extremely myopic eyes often greater than 10 D – referred to as pathologic myopia – the retina is stretched so thin that it is absent in some areas, causing a loss of vision. There may be an associated hemorrhage at the macula, called a Fuchs' spot (Fig. 435).

Another disk variation occurs when the myelin sheath that normally covers the optic nerve

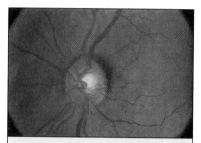

Fig. 433 Normal tigroid (tessellated) fundus with pigment around disk and deeply pigmented choroid.

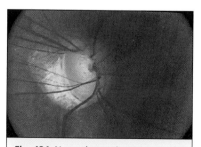

Fig. 434 Normal myopic conus (crescent) at disk margin.

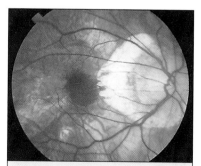

Fig. 435 Pathologic myopia happens most often in eyes with more than 10 D of refractive error.

extends onto the retina, appearing like white flame-shaped patches obscuring the disk margin. It is benign (Fig. 436). The disk margin may also be obscured by drusen (Fig. 437), which are small, round, translucent bodies made up of hyaline deposits that are often calcified. They occur in 0.3–3.7% of eyes. When superficial, they are easy to identify; but when buried, B-scan ultrasound and CT scanning are needed to reveal calcification (see Figs 448 and 449, below). They may damage nerve fibers and cause an enlarged blind spot.

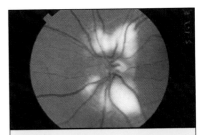

Fig. 436 Myelination of the optic nerve.

Fundus examination

The fundus refers to the inner part of the eye. It is evaluated with an ophthalmoscope. Eye doctors usually dilate the pupils for this exam. Tropicamide (0.5–1%), which relaxes the pupillary sphincter, is preferred because of its quick action (5–10 minutes) and strong effect. Phenylephrine (2.5–10%), which stimulates the dilator muscle, has a weaker effect and takes longer to act (30 minutes). An advantage of phenylephrine is that it doesn't cause the patient's sight to blur as much and won't be as problematic for them when driving home. Both drugs are often used together when more serious retinal disease is suspected.

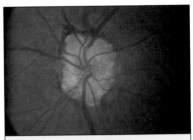

Fig. 437 Disk drusen.

The macula is examined last to minimize miosis and discomfort.

A direct ophthalmoscope (Fig. 438) allows for monocular visualization of the posterior half of the fundus, where most retinal pathology is located. Use a negative lens (red) for myopic eyes and a positive lens (black) for hyperopic eyes. Get as close to the eye as possible and minimize movement by resting the hand that is holding the ophthalmoscope on the patient's cheek, while your other hand lifts the patient's upper lid.

A binocular indirect ophthalmoscope (Fig. 439) consists of a light source worn over the head and a hand-held lens, which allows the entire retina to be seen in three dimensions, albeit upside down. Retinal holes and detachments at the ora serrata can be viewed

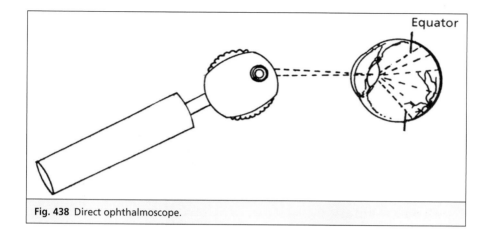

Equator

Fig. 438 Direct ophthalmoscope.

by indenting the sclera with a small thimble worn on the index finger.

A three-mirror contact lens (Fig. 440), used with a slit lamp, gives a detailed stereoscopic view of the entire retina. It is useful in studying subtle changes in each layer of the retina, and to gauge optic cupping. Its disadvantage is the need for anesthetic drops and a gelatinous solution on the eye.

Fluorescein angiography

Fluorescein dye is injected intravenously. As it passes through the retinal circulation, fundus photographs are made in a rapid sequence. This test is useful for evaluating retinal circulation. It demonstrates rate of flow, leakage from capillaries, staining of tissues, areas of nonperfusion, and neovascularization. Retinal blood vessels do not normally leak. Indications for this invasive test may decrease as improvements continually occur in non-invasive optical coherence angiography. See Figs 441 and 442.

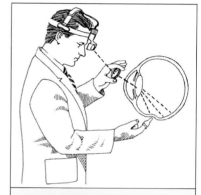

Fig. 439 Indirect ophthalmoscope.

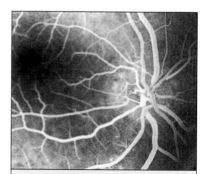

Fig. 441 Normal fluorescein angiogram. Retinal vessels terminate at perifoveal area of the macula. Foveal blood supply comes from underlying choroidal capillaries.

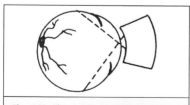

Fig. 440 Three-mirror contact lens.

THE RETINA AND VITREOUS   139

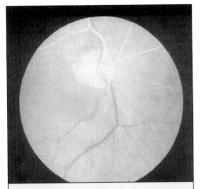

Fig. 442 Fluorescein angiogram of inferior retinal artery occlusion showing lack of perfusion inferiorly after 15.4 seconds.

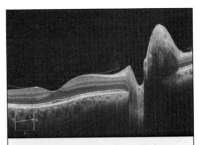

Fig. 443 OCT image of papilledema showing elevated disk margin and hyporeflective (black) areas corresponding to edematous fluid in and around the optic disk. Courtesy of Elizabeth Affel, OCT-C, Wills Eye Hospital.

Papilledema (choked disk)

Papilledema is swelling of the optic nerve specifically due to elevated intracranial pressure that causes a reduction in the ability of fluid to exit the eye. It is usually bilateral and always serious. The intraocular congestion results in a swollen, elevated optic disk with blurred margins. As it progresses, veins become engorged and flame-shaped hemorrhages and cotton-wool spots develop in the peripapillary area.

In 80% of normal eyes there are subtle pulsations of the retinal veins as they exit from the globe at the optic cup. If pulsations are not visible, they can almost always be elicited by exerting slight pressure on the globe (through the lid). In papilledema, one cannot see spontaneous or elicited venous pulsations. Swelling of the optic disk with edema damages the surrounding retina (Figs 443, 445, and 447) enlarging the blind spot (Fig. 446), and is helpful in monitoring the progression or improvement of the disease. The elevated intracranial pressure often causes headache, confusion, nausea, and visual obscurations. Diplopia occurs if the pressure compromises the sixth cranial nerve. Prolonged increased pressure can permanently damage the brain and optic nerve. Common causes are side

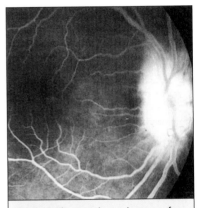

Fig. 444 Fluorescein angiogram of papilledema reveals leakage in and around the optic disk.

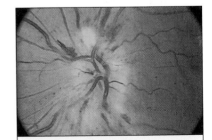

Fig. 445 Papilledema with elevated disk, engorged veins, and flame-shaped hemorrhages.

effects of drugs, such as tetracycline, excessive vitamins, and retinoids used to treat severe acne and psoriasis. Brain tumors, hemorrhages, and infections also could elevate intracranial pressure.

Idiopathic intracranial hypertension (pseudotumor cerebri) is a more common cause of papilledema. It occurs in young, overweight women and may be first discovered by noting papilledema during a routine eye exam (Fig. 445).

Pseudopapilledema

There are many conditions that can mimic the optic disk changes of papilledema and every clue must be considered.

A swollen disk caused by optic neuritis (see Fig. 112) is associated with a Marcus Gunn pupil and loss of central vision, whereas in early papilledema the pupil is normal and there is usually no loss of visual acuity unless edema extends to the macula (Figs 443 and 444) or optic atrophy has already occurred. Early papilledema may be difficult to distinguish from drusen of the disk (Figs 437, 448, and 449) and myelinated nerve fibers (Fig. 436). Both blur the disk margin and cause an enlarged blind spot (Fig. 446). On fluorescein angiography, however, only papilledema has leakage of dye (Fig. 444). A hyperopic

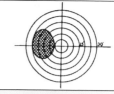

Fig. 446 An enlarged blind spot can be plotted most accurately on a tangent screen. Visual field testing of the size of the blind spot and contraction of the peripheral field must be monitored closely since this is often the only way to know how the papilledema is being controlled, since serial spinal tap pressures are dangerous.

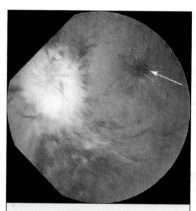

Fig. 447 Papilledema with macular star (↑) due to vitamin A toxicity.

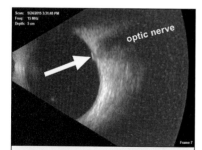

Fig. 448 B-scan ultrasound showing hyperrefective calcification from buried optic disk drusen. Courtesy of Jonathon Prenner, MD, UMDNJ.

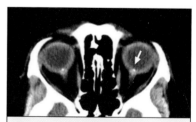

Fig. 449 CT scan performed during workup of what was thought to be papilledema instead revealed calcified optic disk drusen. Courtesy of Elliot Davidoff, MD, Ohio State Medical School.

eye might have a small disk with a blurred margin, but there is no leakage with fluorescein angiography. Like papilledema, central retinal vein occlusion (Fig. 478) may have venous engorgement, a blurred disk margin, and cotton-wool spots. But in central retinal vein occlusion the flame hemorrhages extend out to the peripheral retina and there is more loss of vision. Malignant systemic hypertension (blood pressure 220/120 mmHg) also causes a papilledema-like retinal appearance, which is distinguished by measuring blood pressure on all patients with blurry disk margins (Fig. 454). Orbital diseases decreasing venous outflow from the eye can cause swelling of the disk. Causes include orbital tumors and infections. Idiopathic inflammation of the orbit, also called orbital pseudotumor (Fig. 213), must be considered. Don't confuse orbital pseudotumor with pseudotumor cerebri. In orbital diseases, one looks for localizing signs, such as proptosis. Cavernous sinus disease can also obstruct venous drainage (Figs 76 and 136).

Retinal blood vessels

Retinal vessel walls are normally transparent. They can be visualized because of the blood they contain. In arteriosclerosis, as the vessel walls become hyalinzed, they develop a silver reflex (see Front cover image).

The vessel walls may also whiten when inflamed in conditions such as systemic lupus erythematosus (Fig. 4), sarcoidosis (Fig. 378), cytomegalovirus infection (Figs 390 and 501), and sickle cell disease (Fig. 451). Damaged vessel walls may eventually develop a permanent white sheath and a thread-like lumen. Loss of blood flow, as occurs in retinal artery occlusion, may also cause this change (Fig. 464).

Abnormal capillaries may grow inside the eye in a misguided response to ischemia from retinal artery or vein occlusion and proliferative diabetic retinopathy, most often in and around the optic disk (see Fig. 471). They are due to liberation of vascular endothelial growth factor (VEGF). Panretinal photocoagulation (PRP) may be used to destroy large areas of hypoxic retina, thus decreasing the oxygen demand and the secretion of VEGF. A total of 1500 burns is usually administered to each eye in two sessions (Fig. 450).

Currently there are three anti-VEGF drugs – ranibizumab (Lucentis), bevacizumab (Avastin), and aflibercept (Eylea) – which, when injected into the vitreous, cause regression of the abnormal vessels. They are now being used as a first-line treatment of wet macular degeneration and for macular edema due to retinal vein occlusions and diabetic retinopathy (Figs 494 and 495).

Sickle cell hemoglobinopathy leads to red cells taking on a sickle shape in deoxygenated blood (Figs 451–453). Sickle cell trait (HbAS) affects 8% of African Americans, with 0.4% having sickle cell disease (HbSS) and 0.2% having HbSC disease. Retinal neovascularization resembling "sea fans" occur at the edge of infarcted (pale) areas. Confirm with a sickle cell preparation where a deoxygenating agent is added to the patient's blood. It's positive if red blood cells assume a crescent (sickle) shape.

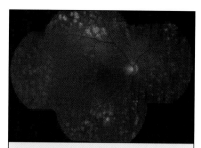

Fig. 450 PRP uses an argon laser to apply 1500 burns to partially destroy retinal tissue while carefully avoiding the central fovea. Also used for proliferative diabetic retinopathy. Courtesy of Daniel Roth, MD, UMDNJ.

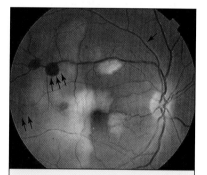

Fig. 451 Sickle cell retinopathy with vascular inflammation (↑), pale areas of ischemic retina salmon-patch intraretinal hemorrhages (↑↑), and pre-retinal hemorrhages (↑↑↑). This occurred in a 26 year-old black male presenting to the emergency department with an acute myocradial infarction, renal failure, and cholecystitis.

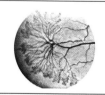

Fig. 452 Sickle cell retinopathy with compensatory neovascularization at edge of infarcted retina. *Source:* S.B. Cohen et al., *Ophthal. Surg.*, 1986, Vol. 17(2), pp. 110–116. Reprinted with permission from SLACK, Inc.

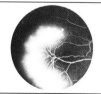

Fig. 453 Fluorescein angiogram showing leakage from abnormal new vessels. *Source:* S.B. Cohen et al., *Ophthal. Surg.*, 1986, Vol. 17(2), pp. 110–116. Reprinted with permission from SLACK, Inc.

Hypertensive retinopathy

Scheie classification		
I	Thinning of retinal arterioles relative to veins	Stages I and II are similar to arteriosclerosis of aging.
II	Obvious arteriolar narrowing with focal areas of attenuation	
III	Stage II, plus cotton-wool spots, exudates, and hemorrhages (Fig. 454)	Stages III and IV are medical emergencies and have strong association with death.
IV	Malignant hypertension, blood pressure 220/120 mmHg	
	Stage III plus swollen optic disk resembling papilledema	

At their junctions, the arteries and veins share a common sheath. As the arteriole wall thickens (arteriosclerosis), it takes on a silvery appearance and causes indentation of the venule, referred to as A-V nicking (Fig. 455). This can lead to a retinal vein occlusion.

Blood pressure	
Normal	<120/80 mmHg
Pre-hypertension	120–139/80–89 mmHg
Hypertension (<60 years)	>140/90 mmHg
Hypertension (>60 years)	>150/90 mmHg
It was shown in a large, 20 year study that half of those treated for hypertension in the USA failed to be controlled.	

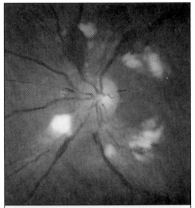

Fig. 454 Stage III hypertensive retinopathy with cotton-wool spots, flame-shaped hemorrhages, and arteriolar narrowing.

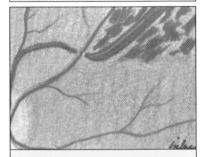

Fig. 455 Drawing of branch retinal vein occlusion with flame hemorrhages and A-V nicking. As the arteriole wall thickens, the A-V crossings change from an acute to a right angle.

Retinal vein occlusion

Retinal vein occlusions cause a painless decrease in vision with hemorrhages extending to the peripheral retina (Fig. 478). Acutely, there are flame-shaped hemorrhages and dot-and-blot hemorrhages (Figs 455 and 456) which may last for years. Cotton-wool spots and a poorly reactive pupil usually indicate an ischemic retina and are more ominous. Ischemia is confirmed with fluorescein angiography or OCT angiography (OCTA; Figs 459–461). One half of the ischemic cases stimulate secretion of VEGF, causing new blood vessel growth on the iris which can bleed and lead to glaucoma. Not all new vessels are bad. Late-onset, tortuous, retino-choroidal, collateral vessels could develop on the optic disk, and elsewhere on the retina, and are beneficial in helping the obstructed venous blood exit the eye via the choroidal route (Fig. 457). If macular edema occurs, it may be treated with localized laser to the retina, monthly intravitreal injections of anti-VEGF or steroid (Fig. 495). There are corticosteroid intravitreal implants that provide a prolonged, slow release. Therapy continues until OCT reveals resolution of edema. Treatment should also address the frequently associated risk factors such as hypertension, dyslipidemia, diabetes, and hypercoagulability.

Spectral domain OCT (SD-OCT) is a noninvasive office imaging device. OCT images are created by measuring reflected light. Images may be produced in color or black and white. The latter is preferred because of the increased detail. Low reflectivity appears as black, optically empty space and occurs within a normal vitreous and in cystic areas containing serous fluid and edema. High reflectivity appears white as with solid membranes (Fig. 458), blood, drusen, RPE, choroidal nevi, and scars. Resolution to as little as 3 μm has allowed the study of tissues almost to a cellular level. It is used to discern fluid within the layers of the retina especially with respect to macular edema (Figs 443, 458–460, 465, 468, and 490–492). It is also helpful in evaluating the vitreoretinal interface (Fig. 537), macular holes (Figs 537–540), age-related macular degeneration (AMD; Figs 490–492), and epiretinal membranes (Figs 524–528). OCTA measures reflections from moving blood and has an advantage over fluorescein angiography because it is non-invasive and can distinguish vessels in the superficial or deep retina and the choroid (Figs 461, 473–476, and 492).

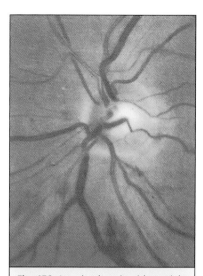

Fig. 456 Arteriosclerosis with partial vein occlusion causing engorged vein inferiorly and a secondary flame hemorrhage. "Silver wire" changes are noted at the superior disk margin.

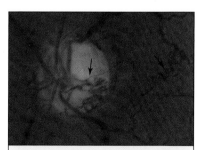

Fig. 457 Central retinal vein occlusion 3 months after occurrence. Collateral curlicue vessels on the disk and retina (↑) help venous blood exit the eye. They don't bleed or leak fluorescein as do new blood vessels in diabetes. Courtesy of Julia Monsonego, CRA, Wills Eye Hospital.

1. Internal Limiting Membrane	
2. Posterior Cortical Vitreous	
3. Preretinal Space	
4. Nerve Fiber Layer	
5. Ganglion Cell Layer	
6. Inner Plexiform Layer	
7. Inner Nuclear Layer	
8. Outer Plexiform Layer	
9.1. Henle Fiber Layer	
9.2. Outer Nuclear layer	
10. External Limiting Membrane	
11. Myoid Zone	
12. Inner Segment / Outer Segment Junction or Ellipsoid Zone	
13. Outer Segments of Photoreceptors	
14. Interdigitation Zone	
15. RPE / Bruch's Complex	
16. Choriocapillaris	
17. Sattler's Layer (Small choroidal vessels)	
18. Haller's Layer (Large choroidal vessels)	
19. Choroid Sclera Junction	

Fig. 458 OCT of normal macula. Courtesy of Carl Zeiss Meditec, Inc.

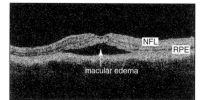

Fig. 459 Colored OCT of macular edema after retinal vein occlusion. Measurement of decreasing retinal thickness together with improvement of vision is used to monitor the response to treatment. RPE, retinal pigment epithelium; NFL, nerve fiber layer.

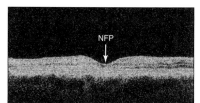

Fig. 460 OCT of resolved macular edema from retinal vein occlusion after intravitreal triamcinolone injection. Vision improved from 20/400 to 20/30. NFP, normal foveal pit. Courtesy of Jennifer Hancock.

Retinal artery occlusion

Retinal artery occlusion (Figs 442, 462–465, and 543) causes sudden, painless, loss of vision. Carotid artery plaques (Figs 135 and 545–547) or heart disease such as arrhythmias, endocarditis, or valve abnormalities may liberate fine platelets or larger cholesterol emboli (Hollenhorst plaque), which lodge in arterial bifurcations. Sludging of blood flow gives a box-car appearance (Fig. 463). Some irreparable loss of vision usually occurs within 1 hour, and the loss is almost impossible to reverse after 12 hours. Eventually, optic atrophy results (Fig. 464). Any ocular treatment is of questionable value. You could have the patient breathe into a paper bag to elevate CO_2, which dilates the artery; or lower the eye pressure with oral or topical medications. Gently massaging the eye may

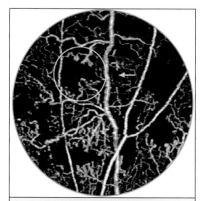

Fig. 461 OCTA of branch retinal vein occlusion with engorged vein (↑) and adjacent ischemic area of non-perfusion. Courtesy of Carl Zeiss Meditec, Inc.

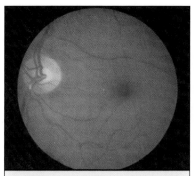

Fig. 462 Retinal artery occlusion with a cholesterol Hollenhorst plaque on disk and a cherry-red spot in the fovea where choroidal blood is seen outlined by a swollen ischemic macula.

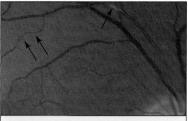

Fig. 463 Branch retinal artery occlusion with embolus (↑) and sludging of blood (box-car effect, ↑↑) due to a decreased flow. Courtesy of Julia Monsonego, CRA, Wills Eye Hospital.

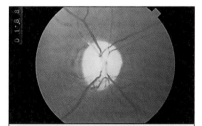

Fig. 464 Late-stage retinal artery occlusion with optic atrophy and arteries that are thread-like and sheathed.

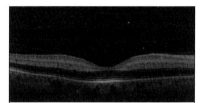

Fig. 465 OCT of central retinal artery occlusion with inner retinal layer thickening due to cloudy swelling and a hyporeflective outer layer due to edema. Courtesy of David Yarian, MD, UMDNJ.

get the embolus to move on. Call an eye doctor immediately to tap the anterior chamber, which further lowers eye pressure. Refer the patient to a neurologist as soon as possible, since it is not uncommon for a second stroke elsewhere in the following weeks.

Diabetic retinopathy

Half of US adults have diabetes or pre-diabetes, the latter characterized by a glycated hemoglobin A_1c (HbA$_1$c) level of 5.7–6.4% and fasting glucose levels of 100–125 mg/dL. In patients with diabetes there is an HbA$_1$c level greater than 6.5% and a fasting plasma glucose level of 126 mg/dL or greater, or a 2 hour post-prandial glucose level greater than 200 mg/dL (see table, p. 150).

Type 1 diabetes (insulin-dependent) is due to decreased secretion of insulin by the B-cells in the pancreas and is largely caused by an auto-immune process. Type 2 diabetes (adult onset) is primarily due to cellular resistance to insulin. Type 2 accounts for 90% of diabetes and is often related to obesity and lack of exercise. Both types cause elevated blood sugar with damage to the microvasculature of the retina.

There are three progressive stages of diabetic retinopathy (see Front cover image) that often begin to appear in 25% of eyes after 10 years, 50% after 15 years, and 80% after 20 years. These percentages vary depending on control of blood sugar and lifestyle changes.

Stage 1 Non-proliferative or background retinopathy is a microvascular breakdown in the blood–retina barrier, causing leakage of plasma and lipid. It initially presents with microaneurysms, dot hemorrhages, and white exudates at the macula (see Front cover image and Fig. 466). This is the most common reason for loss of vision in diabetic retinopathy. The macular edema (Figs 467 and 468) is usually treated with focal laser photocoagulation, intravitreal injection of triamcinolone (steroid), or anti-VEGF.

Stage 2 Preproliferative retinopathy (Fig. 469) is due to widespread capillary closure (Figs 471 and 473–476) causing retinal ischemia. There are cotton-wool spots, venous beading, blot hemorrhages, and the absence of blood flow on fluorescein angiography (see Fig. 470 and Front cover image).

Stage 3 Proliferative diabetic retinopathy occurs when the ischemic areas of the retina stimulate the growth of abnormal curlicue

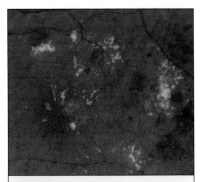

Fig. 466 Stage 1: background retinopathy with microaneurysms, exudates, and dot hemorrhages. Courtesy of Julia Monsonego, CRA, Wills Eye Hospital.

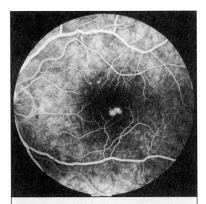

Fig. 467 Leakage of fluorescein from microaneurysms. Normal retinal vessels do not leak.

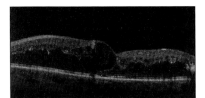

Fig. 468 OCT of diffuse diabetic macular edema with hyporeflective (black) retinal thickening giving spongey appearance. Courtesy of David Yarian, MD, UMDNJ.

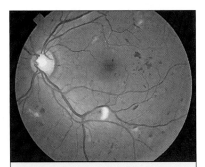

Fig. 469 Stage 2: preproliferative retinopathy with cotton-wool spots, microaneurysms, and dot hemorrhages.

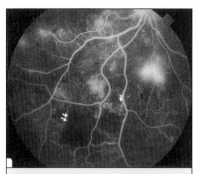

Fig. 470 Fluorescein angiogram showing neovascularization (↓) adjacent to dark area of capillary nonperfusion (↓↓).

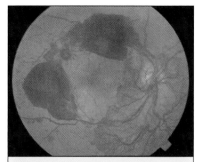

Fig. 471 Stage 3a: proliferative retinopathy with neovascularization and pre-retinal hemorrhages.

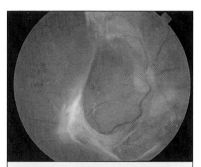

Fig. 472 Stage 3b: fibrous proliferation. These membranes may contract and cause a retinal detachment.

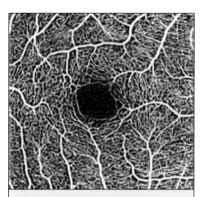

Fig. 473 Normal black and white OCTA. Note ring of interconnected capillaries at the margin of the avascular fovea. Courtesy of Carl Zeiss Meditec, Inc.

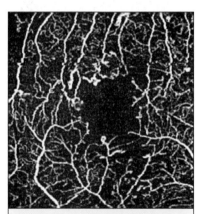

Fig. 474 Black and white OCTA of diabetic retinopathy showing microaneurysms and area of ischemia appearing as darkened areas of non-perfusion. Courtesy of Carl Zeiss Meditec, Inc.

capillaries on the surface of the retina, most often around the disk and on the iris (Figs 359 and 360). The former may grow into a vitreous bleed and totally obstruct vision and the view of the retina. They then can cause fibrotic membranes (Fig. 472) that contract, resulting in retinal detachments. PRP (Fig. 450) destroys part of the oxygen-demanding retina, thus reducing the release of VEGF that causes neovascularization. In PRP, 1500 argon laser burns are given in two sessions, often causing regression of neovascularization within several weeks. Intravitreal injection of anti-VEGF also causes regression of new vessels. This third stage occurs late in the course of diabetes and is associated with other serious systemic vascular changes and an associated 56% 5 year survival rate. Diabetics should see an eye doctor annually for a retina examination through a dilated pupil, although children may be exempt in the first years of diabetes.

To minimize these changes, one should ideally keep fasting blood sugar below 110 mg/dL, blood pressure less than 130/80 mmHg (10 mmHg less than non-diabetics), exercise, stay thin, reduce abdominal obesity, and keep HbA_1c levels below 6.5%, although lower levels are even better. HbA_1c gives an estimate of the preceding 2–3 months' control of blood sugar. For each additional percentage point of HbA_1c there is a 50% increase in

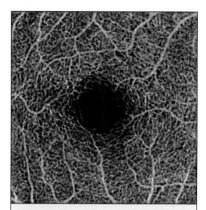

Fig. 475 Normal color (OCTA) of perifoveal retina. Superficial retinal vessels are red; deep retinal vessels are green. Courtesy of Carl Zeiss Meditec, Inc.

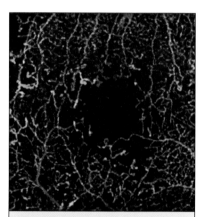

Fig. 476 Diabetic retinopathy imaged with color OCTA showing microaneurysms and darkened ischemic areas of retinal capillary non-perfusion (compare with Fig. 475). Courtesy of Carl Zeiss Meditec, Inc.

Approximate equivalent	
HbA_1c (%)	Mean non-fasting glucose (mg/dL)
4	65
5	100
6	135
7	170
8	205
9.5	226
10.0	240
10.5	255
11.0	269
11.5	283

Depth of retinal hemorrhages

Preretinal hemorrhages

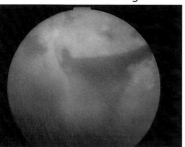

Fig. 477 Pre-retinal hemorrhages lie between the retina internal limiting membrane and the posterior hyaloid surface of the vitreous. They may layer out to a boat shape. Common causes include a proliferative diabetic retinopathy, trauma, vitreous detachments, and leukemia (Fig. 482). This blood could break into the vitreous and obscure the view.

Superficial hemorrhages

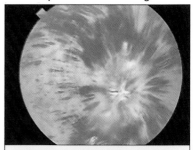

Fig. 478 This central retinal vein occlusion shows superficial flame-shaped hemorrhages that follow the contour of the nerve fiber layer and radiate from the optic disk far out into the periphery. Flame hemorrhages also occur in papilledema, diabetes, hypertension, and optic neuritis, but do not extend to the peripheral retina as in central retinal vein occlusion.

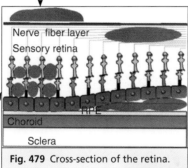

Nerve fiber layer
Sensory retina
RPE
Choroid
Sclera

Fig. 479 Cross-section of the retina.

Deep retinal hemorrhages

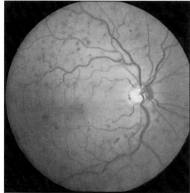

Fig. 480 Intraretinal hemorrhages in partial central retinal vein occlusion.

Subretinal hemorrhages

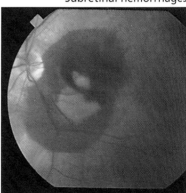

Fig. 481 Wet macular degeneration with subretinal hemorrhages that are greyish in appearance since they are under the RPE. The red hemorrhages broke into the deep retina.

complications of diabetes. By lowering systolic blood pressure by 10 mmHg there could be a 40% reduction in retinopathy. A small number of non-diabetics may also develop a mild form of retinopathy resembling diabetic retinopathy, indicating that there may be factors other than plasma glucose levels responsible for these changes.

Age-related macular degeneration

Age-related macular degeneration (AMD) occurs after age 50 and is the leading cause of blindness in elderly persons. Twenty-five percent of 70 year-old people have signs of the condition, and this number increases to 50% by age 90. The main symptom is loss of central vision. In a normal retina (Fig. 483), the RPE has tight junctions protecting the sensory retina from leakage of more permeable choroidal capillaries. The RPE also metabolically supports the rods and cones, concentrating the vitamin A needed to regenerate the visual pigment rhodopsin and creating an adhesive force with the overlying neurosensory retina, which prevents retinal detachments.

There are two types of AMD. The more common, the dry non-vascular type, accounts for 90% of cases. In dry AMD, Bruch's membrane degenerates by fragmenting in some areas and thickening with hyaline (drusen) in other areas (Figs 484, 485, 502, and 504). There is

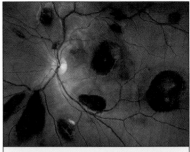

Fig. 482 White centered pre-retinal hemorrhages called Roth spots may occur in anemia, leukemia, and bacterial endocartitis. Courtesy of Debra Brown, COT, CRA, University of San Francisco.

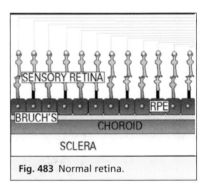

Fig. 483 Normal retina.

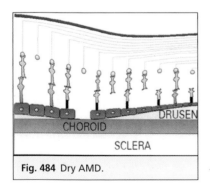

Fig. 484 Dry AMD.

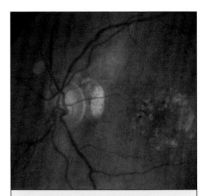

Fig. 485 Dry AMD with pigment mottling, drusen, and loss of the foveal reflex. Courtesy of Elliot Davidoff, MD.

often pigment mottling and loss of the foveal reflex. The RPE on top of the drusen degenerates. The overlying sensory retina, which is metabolically dependent on the RPE, thins out, resulting in atrophic macular degeneration. If enough retina disappears, the underlying choroidal vasculature is easily visualized with an ophthalmoscope. Advanced dry AMD is termed geographic AMD or geographic atrophy (Fig. 486) because of the large circumscribed atrophic areas through which choroidal vessels can be seen.

Dry AMD may be treated with supplements of vitamins A, E, and C, zinc, lutein, zeaxanthin, and omega-3 fatty acids. These are available in various combinations over the counter. These supplements reduce loss of vision by 25%. Avoiding cigarettes and wearing ultraviolet protective lenses is also beneficial.

About 10% of the dry AMD may progress to the wet type in which choroidal blood vessels (subretinal neovascularization) form (Figs 487–492). The goal is to recognize these vessels before they bleed and cause a hemorrhagic detachment of the RPE, which appears dark red. When they penetrate Bruch's membrane and the sensory retina they appear bright red (Fig. 488). Eventually, the blood could fibrose and form a white scar (Fig. 493), called disciform macular degeneration. An early symptom of progression from the dry to wet form may be that straight lines become wavy on the Amsler grid. The patient may monitor at home (see Figs 124 and 551).

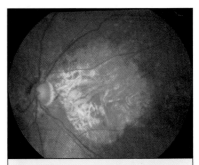

Fig. 486 The advanced dry AMD is called geographic AMD. The thinned RPE exposes underlying choroidal vasculature. Courtesy of Elliot Davidoff, MD.

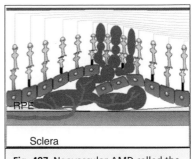

Fig. 487 Neovascular AMD called the wet type.

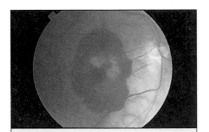

Fig. 488 Hemorrhagic stage of wet AMD may be associated with severe vision loss and fibrous scarring.

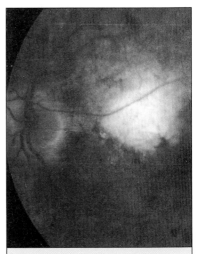

Fig. 489 Fluorescein angiogram of subretinal neovascular membrane.

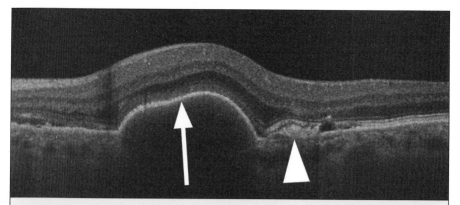

Fig. 490 OCT of wet AMD with increased retinal thickening due to edema (appears black); pigment epithelial detachment (↑) with significant elevation; penetration of pigment epithelial layer by choroidal vessels (∧). Courtesy of David Yarian, MD, UMDNJ.

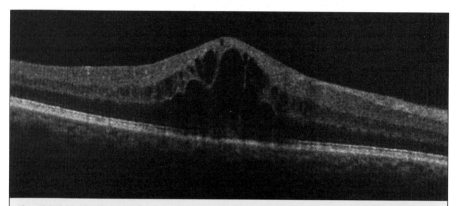

Fig. 491 OCT of wet AMD with cystoid macular edema. This loculated type of edema also occurs in diabetes, retinal vein occlusions, uveitis, and most commonly in 2–60% of cataract surgeries during the post-operative period.

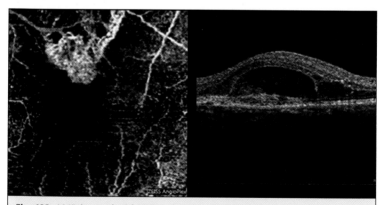

Fig. 492 AMD imaged with OCTA showing choroidal neovascularization. Courtesy of Carl Zeiss Meditec, Inc.

The initial treatment for wet AMD is a monthly or bimonthly (every 2 months) intra-vitreal injection of an anti-VEGF such as ran-ibizumab (Lucentis), bevacizumab (Avastin), or aflibercept (Eylea) (Figs 494 and 495) for an as-yet-undetermined – perhaps indefinite – number of months. This drug antagonizes VEGF, causing regression of abnormal vessels.

If anti-VEGF therapy is not effective, laser photodynamic therapy may be used. Intra-venously administered verteporfin (Visu-dyne) concentrates in the choroidal vascu-lature. A low-energy laser is then aimed at the vessels, activating the dye, causing most cell death inside the vessel, but also some collateral retinal damage. Laser is usually reserved for non-central edema that is far enough away from the fovea to minimize loss of vision. Besides wet AMD, Visudyne/laser therapy is used to treat choroidal neo-vascularization in pathologic myopia and histoplasmosis (Fig. 380). Intravitreal triam-cinolone (steroid) injection may be added to reduce inflammation.

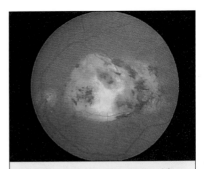

Fig. 493 Late-stage wet AMD with disciform scar following hemorrhage.

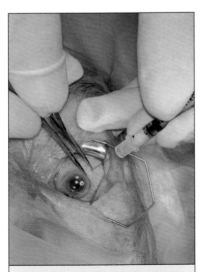

Fig. 494 Pars plana injection of an anti-VEGF to treat wet AMD. Calipers measure a site 3.5 mm posterior to limbus in the space between the retina and vascular ciliary body. Courtesy of Elliot Davidoff, MD.

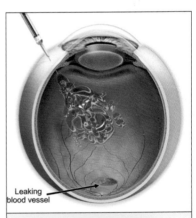

Leaking blood vessel

Fig. 495 Intravitreal injections are becoming the most common intraocular ophthalmic procedure performed in the USA, doubling that of cataract surgery. Besides anti-VEGF, which is the most common medication injected into the vitreous, others include the steroids triamcinolone and dexamethasone; the antivirals ganciclovir and foscarnet, used to treat herpes and cytomegalovirus; the antibiotics vancomycin, ceftazidime, and amikacin; and the antifungal amphotericin B.

Rarer forms and causes of macular degeneration are juvenile inherited types, such as Stargardt's disease (the most common); chorioretinitis; infection; and staring at the sun. Reassure patients that they never go totally blind, but only lose central vision, often resulting in 20/400 vision.

Central serous chorioretinopathy

Central serous chorioretinopathy (Figs 496–499) is a macular disease in which a defect in the RPE allows choroidal fluid to leak into the sensory retina. The incidence is six times higher in men, often aged 25–40, and may be triggered by corticosteroids and stress. Symptoms are decreased and distorted vision. Wavy lines are demonstrated with an Amsler grid (Fig. 551). Ophthalmoscopically, it is difficult to visualize the clear, oval elevation of the retina. It is easily diagnosed with fluorescein angiography (Fig. 497) or the less invasive OCT (Fig. 499). Eighty to ninety percent clear within a few months. Photodynamic laser therapy may be used if leakage continues for 6 months.

Pseudoxanthoma elasticum

Pseudoxanthoma elasticum is a systemic disease. There may be cardiovascular abnormalities, gastrointestinal hemorrhages, and loose skin folds on the neck (Fig. 506). On fundus exam, there are angioid streaks (Fig. 505), which also occur in Ehlers–Danlos, Paget's, and sickle cell disease.

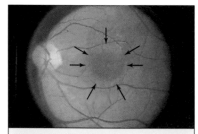

Fig. 496 Central serous chorioretinopathy.

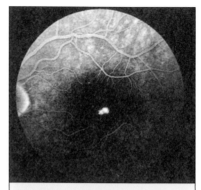

Fig. 497 Fluorescein leakage through the RPE in central serous chorioretinopathy, often appearing as a single "smoke stack."

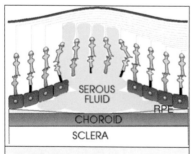

Fig. 498 Central serous chorioretinopathy.

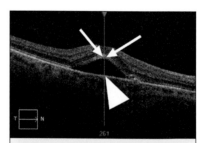

Fig. 499 OCT of central serous chorioretinopathy showing subretinal fluid; pigmented epithelial detachments (elevations) (↑↑) and thickening of the choriocapillaries with thinning of the RPE (^). Courtesy of David Yarian, MD, UMDNJ.

White and yellow retinal lesions

Cotton-wool spots

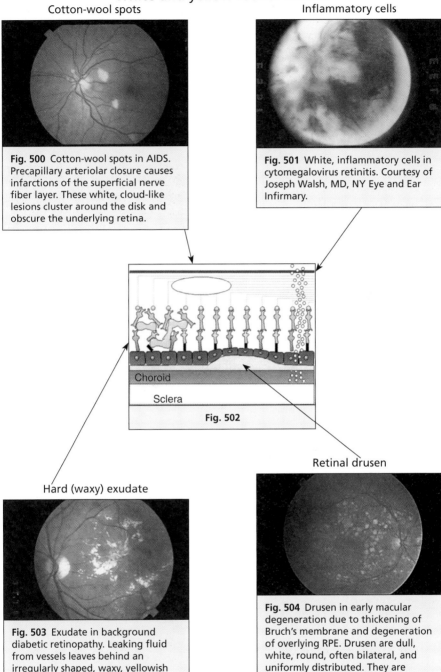

Fig. 500 Cotton-wool spots in AIDS. Precapillary arteriolar closure causes infarctions of the superficial nerve fiber layer. These white, cloud-like lesions cluster around the disk and obscure the underlying retina.

Inflammatory cells

Fig. 501 White, inflammatory cells in cytomegalovirus retinitis. Courtesy of Joseph Walsh, MD, NY Eye and Ear Infirmary.

Choroid

Sclera

Fig. 502

Hard (waxy) exudate

Fig. 503 Exudate in background diabetic retinopathy. Leaking fluid from vessels leaves behind an irregularly shaped, waxy, yellowish lipoprotein residue. It is seen most often in diabetes and retinal vein occlusions.

Retinal drusen

Fig. 504 Drusen in early macular degeneration due to thickening of Bruch's membrane and degeneration of overlying RPE. Drusen are dull, white, round, often bilateral, and uniformly distributed. They are sometimes hard to distinguish from waxy exudates that are yellow and irregular in shape and distribution.

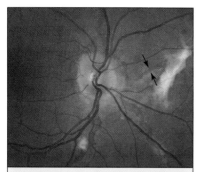

Fig. 505 Pseudoxanthoma elasticum: angloid streaks are breaks in Bruch's membrane (↑) that radiate from the peripapillary area. Courtesy of Julia Monsonego, CRA, Wills Eye Hospital.

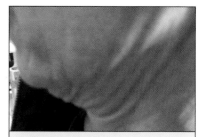

Fig. 506 Don't confuse pseudoxanthoma elasticum and Ehlers–Danlos (ED) syndrome. Both are inherited diseases of the skin elasticity (loose skin on the neck), arterial aneurysms, blue sclera, and retinal angioid streaks. Unique to Ehlers–Danlos is hyperextensibility of the joints.

Albinism

Albinism has many forms and refers to inherited hypopigmentation. Common findings in all types involving the eye are photophobia, hypopigmentation of the retina (Fig. 507), and transillumination of the iris with a penlight at the limbus (Fig. 508). Additional findings may include nystagmus, a hypoplastic macula with absence of a foveal reflex, reduced vision, refractive errors, decreased immunity, and decreased pigmentation of the hair and skin (Fig. 509).

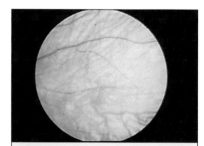

Fig. 507 Albinotic fundus.

Retinitis pigmentosa

Retinitis pigmentosa (Figs 510–513) is a slowly progressive hereditary rod and cone degeneration. Inheritance patterns include autosomal dominant or recessive and X-linked recessive. Since it begins in the retinal periphery, the first loss is peripheral and night vision, often sparing central visual acuity for many years. The retina has pigmentary changes resembling bone corpuscles. The diagnosis is confirmed with an electroretinogram.

Researchers have restored some vision in humans with implantation of silicon microchips in the subretinal or epiretinal space to

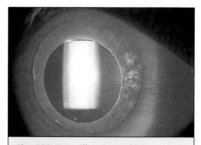

Fig. 508 Transilluminated iris.

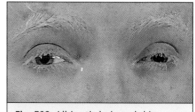

Fig. 509 Albinotic hair and skin.

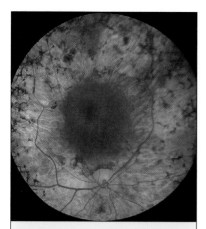

Fig. 510 Retinitis pigmentosa with boney pigmented spicules. Courtesy of John Fingert, MD, and *Arch. Ophthalmol.*, Sept. 2008, Vol. 126, No. 9, pp. 1301–1303.

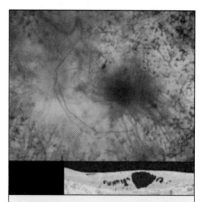

Fig. 511 Retinitis pigmentosa with macular cyst clearly visible on OCT. Courtesy of Alexis Smith, CRA, OCT-C, Kellogg Eye Center, Ann Arbor, MI.

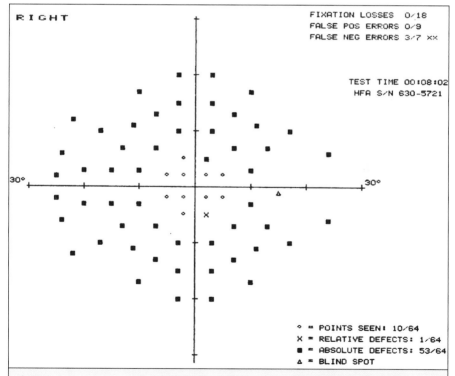

Fig. 512 Constricted visual field in late-stage retinitis pigmentosa. Dark squares indicate absence of vision.

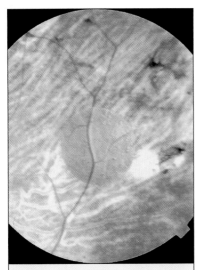

Fig. 513 A microchip in the subretinal space (note black pigment clumping typical of retinitis pigmentosa). Courtesy of Alan and Vincent Chow.

convert light energy into electrical current (Fig. 513). The Argus II epiretinal prosthesis was recently approved by the US Food and Drug Administration.

Retinoblastoma

This is a malignant tumor of the retina, often appearing by 2 years of age. Most arise from a genetic mutation that survivors may transmit in a Mendelian dominant fashion. There may be one or more white, elevated retinal masses which are bilateral 30% of the time (Fig. 514). A CT scan often reveals calcifications in the tumor. In the past, enucleation (Fig. 394) was a primary treatment. Now attempts at salvaging some vision and the globe are replacing enucleation with injection of chemotherapeutic agents into the ophthalmic artery, radiation therapy, laser therapy, cryotherapy, and intravitreal chemo-injections. All infants at 3 and 6 months should be tested for a red pupillary reflex, which should reveal symmetric red reflections with no opacities (Fig. 515).

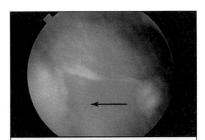

Fig. 514 Retinoblastoma. Courtesy of David Taylor.

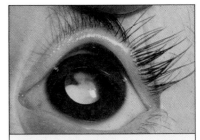

Fig. 515 Leukocoria (white pupil) due to retinoblastoma.

Retinopathy of prematurity

Retinopathy of prematurity (ROP) is a disease of newborns that occurs in premature infants weighing less than 1500 g or having a gestational age of 28 weeks or less. It occurs more often when oxygen is administered.

Normal vascularization of the retina progresses peripherally and is not normally completed until 1 month after birth. Oxygen given to newborns stops this normal vascularization process. When the oxygen is discontinued, the avascular peripheral retina stimulates new vessel growth (Figs 516 and 517). These new vessels, however, are now abnormal and may bleed, resulting in vitreous hemorrhage with fibrous proliferation. It can drag the retina (Fig. 518), sometimes causing a retinal detachment. The ideal therapy is comprehensive prenatal care to reduce the number of premature births and careful monitoring of oxygen in the nursery.

ROP is becoming more prevalent because of advances in neonatal intensive care, which have lead to an improvement in survival for very low birthweight infants. An eye doctor should check the peripheral retina at 6 weeks of chronological age or 32 weeks' gestational age, which was earlier.

Laser photocoagulation, or less often transscleral cryotherapy, may be used to scar the avascular retina in stage 3 when the demarcation line is elevated with fibrovascular proliferation. Rigid examination and treatment guidelines and frequent poor visual outcomes are causing a shortage of doctors willing to follow these infants and be exposed to high-cost litigation. A web-based telemedicine system is presently being evaluated. Retinal photographs taken by nurses and technicians are being sent to remote sites to be reviewed by experts.

Vitreous

The vitreous is a clear gel that is 98% water. The viscosity is due to hyaluronic acid and

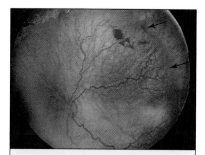

Fig. 516 Stage 3 retinopathy of prematurity (ROP). Note line of demarcation where normal retinal vessels stopped growing (↑). It is initially a flat line (stage 1), then it forms a ridge (stage 2) before abnormal vessels start growing (stage 3). Laser treatment will hopefully prevent a stage 4 retinal detachment.

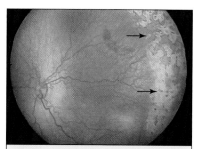

Fig. 517 Regression of abnormal vessels and hemorrhages after treating ischemic peripheral retina with laser (↑). Courtesy of Anna L. Ellis, MD, and *Arch. Ophthalmol.*, Oct. 2002, Vol. 120, p. 1405. Copyright 2002, American Medical Association. All rights reserved.

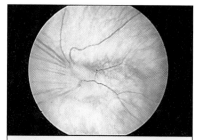

Fig. 518 Late stage of retinopathy of prematurity with disk and retinal vessels dragged peripherally.

collagen fibrils. It fills the interior of the globe like air fills a balloon.

Disorders in the retina and choroid often cause debris to be deposited in this clear gel. The patient perceives the changes as shifting floaters, especially evident when viewing a bright white surface. A recent onset of this symptom requires a dilated retina examination with an indirect ophthalmoscope.

White cells in the vitreous (Fig. 519) are found in uveitis, endophthalmitis, or papillitis. Red cells occur most often from hemorrhages associated with diabetic retinopathy. Retinal holes, detachments, and trauma are less common causes (Figs 520 and 521).

In asteroid hyalosis, hundreds of small, spherical balls are suspended in the vitreous and, amazingly, aren't very annoying to the patient. When questioned, they admit to seeing floaters (Fig. 522). These calcium phospholipid crystals deposit in the vitreous for no apparent reason. Ophthalmoscopically, these appear like stars in the galaxy and are benign, requiring no treatment.

B-scan ultrasound can be useful in evaluation of the retina when direct visualization is obscured by blood cells in the vitreous, cataracts, or corneal opacities.

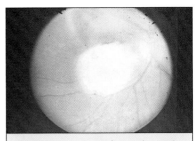

Fig. 519 Hazy view of toxoplasmosis choroiditis due to white cells in the vitreous.

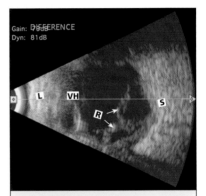

Fig. 520 B-scan ultrasound of retinal detachment (R) with vitreous hemorrhage (VH), posterior surface of lens (L), and sclera (S).

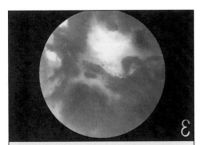

Fig. 521 Blunt trauma, causing pre-, intra-, and subretinal hemorrhage is referred to as a commotio retinae. Hemorrhage may extend into the vitreous. Traumatic hemorrhages also occur in 85% of cases of shaken-baby syndrome and must be looked for when physical abuse is suspected.

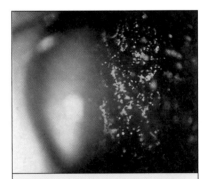

Fig. 522 Slit lamp view of asteroid hyalosis with lens seen on left and vitreous on right.

Posterior vitreous detachment

The vitreous normally liquefies and shrinks with age with a prevalence of 63% in people over 70 (Fig. 523). It is most strongly adherent to the retina at the vitreous base (near the ora serrata), the macula, and the optic disk. Traction on these areas can normally cause some flashing lights and floaters with no consequences. However, posterior vitreous detachment (PVD) could tear the very thin superficial internal limiting membrane (ILM) covering the nerve fiber layer of the retina.

Breaks in the ILM allow glial cells to grow onto the surface of the retina. These epiretinal membranes (ERMs) occur in 34% of adults over 63 years of age. This gliosis at first is a clear, glistening, cellophane-like membrane that can then progress to a more translucent, and then opaque, membrane that can reduce vision. The ERM can contract and cause macular pucker with wrinkling of the retina and distortion of vision (Figs 524 and 525). If vision is significantly affected, surgical vitrectomy and membranectomy can be performed (Figs 526–528).

In 12% of cases of PVD the tear is more severe than just the ILM and extends partway (Fig. 538) through the sensory retina. Of these partial retinal holes, 70% go on to develop into full-thickness holes (Fig. 539) or even a retinal detachment (Fig. 529).

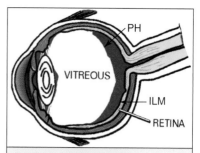

Fig. 523 Posterior vitreous detachment. The posterior surface of the vitreous is called the posterior hyaloid (PH) and is made up of condensed collagen fibers. The membrane covering the adjacent retinal surface is called the internal limiting membrane (ILM).

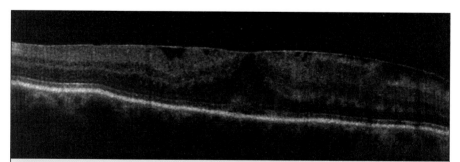

Fig. 524 OCT of epiretinal membrane appearing as white line on surface of the retina. Contraction causing pucker due to wrinkling and thickening of retina from macular edema. Courtesy of David Yarian, MD, UMDNJ.

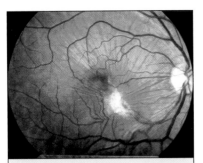

Fig. 525 Macular pucker with visible traction lines It occurs in 6% of the population.

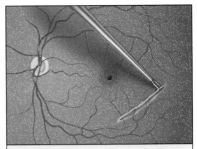

Fig. 526 A blade or forceps is used to create an initial flap in the internal limiting membrane. Triamcinolone crystals may be injected to coat the membrane for easier identifications. Illustration by Chris Gralapp.

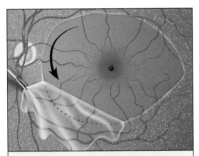

Fig. 527 A circular tear then peels the opacified epithelial membrane with or without the ILM. Illustration by Chris Gralapp.

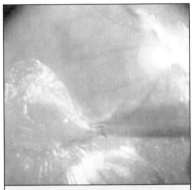

Fig. 528 Peeling of epiretinal membrane. *Source*: M.E. Parah, M. Maia, and E.B. Rodrigues, *Am. J. Ophthalmol.*, 2009, Vol. 148(3), p. 338. Reproduced with permission of Elsevier.

Retinal holes and detachments

A retinal detachment (or RD) is a separation of the neurosensory retina containing the rods and cones from the underlying RPE (Fig. 529). There is normally a low-grade adhesion between these two layers, which can be broken by traction or fluid entering the space between them. Sixty-six percent of retinal detachments begin with myopic thinning of lattice degeneration in the peripheral retina. Lattice degeneration is seen with an indirect ophthalmoscope in 8% of eyes as a white meshwork of lines with black pigment near the ora serrata (Figs 530 and 532). Holes may develop in these areas spontaneously or from trauma, cataract surgery, vitreous traction (Fig. 537),

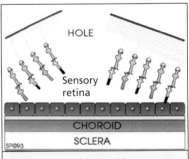

Fig. 529 Retinal hole with detachment of sensory retina from pigment epithelium.

or contraction of diabetic retinal membranes. Fluid enters the holes and detaches the retina (Figs 531 and 532). This is called rhegmatogenous retinal detachment. Not all holes cause problems. Small, round, asymptomatic holes may often be left untreated. Large horseshoe holes with vitreous traction and recent symptoms must be sealed. Less frequently occurring is a non-rhegmatogenous retinal detachment with no holes, which may be due to choroidal effusions into the retina as occurs with choroidal tumors and scleritis. Symptoms of retinal detachment often include loss of vision, described as a "curtain," with flashes and floaters. Ophthalmoscopically, it appears as an elevated, grey membrane unless a vitreous hemorrhage obscures it. Fine, reddish vitreous debris ("tobacco dust") liberated by the RPE may be seen with a slit lamp and should alert one to a possible retinal hole or detachment.

Surgical repair of the hole using laser therapy, cryotherapy, or diathermy creates a chorioretinal adhesive scar (Fig. 533). Treatment is most urgent when the macula has not yet been

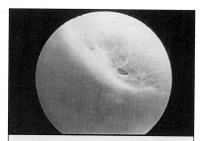

Fig. 530 Lattice degeneration with round hole. Courtesy of Leo Bores.

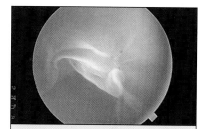

Fig. 531 Retinal detachment with large hole.

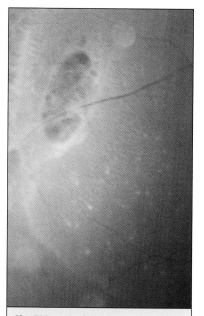

Fig. 532 Retinal detachment caused by large tear and hole in area of lattice degeneration.

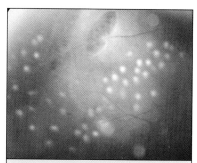

Fig. 533 After cryotherapy, the retinal detachment in the figure above is treated with the expansile gas C_3F_8, and positioning of the body so that the bubble tamponades the tear. Courtesy of Jiuhn-Feng Hwang, MD, and San-Ni Chen, MD. Reprinted from *Am. J. Ophthalmol.*, Feb. 2007, Vol. 143, No. 2, pp. 217–221, with permission from Elsevier.

affected. Depending on the type and size of the detachment, increasingly, more complex surgery may be done. Small holes and detachments, especially at the 12 o'clock position, can be repaired with pneumatic retinopexy where a gas is injected into the vitreous. It presses the retina against the choroid and tamponades the hole by manipulating the patient's head position. Air is often used and is absorbed in several days. The expansive gas perfluropropate (C_3F_8), when needed, lasts for weeks. Silicone oil is used in more complicated cases and is removed in 2–3 months. A pars plana vitrectomy is done if vitreoretinal traction is suspected. An encircling scleral buckle (Figs 534 and 535) pushes the sclera against the retina. In this case, subretinal fluid is drained through a scleral incision and cryotherapy or diathermy is applied to the retina through the sclera.

Vitreomacular traction could resolve on its own by spontaneous lysis of the adhesion, or it can lead to macular cysts and partial- or full-thickness holes. Partial-thickness holes (lamellar holes) can partially reduce vision and may be observed without treatment (Fig. 538). However, 70% may progress to full thickness with severe loss of central vision and should be monitored. A vitrectomy may be performed to release traction bands (Figs 537, 539–542). Air is then injected into the vitreous space and the patient is sent home to lie on their stomach for 2 weeks so that the air rises and

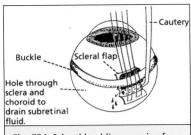
Fig. 534 Scleral buckling repair of retinal detachment.

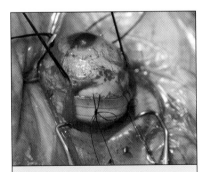
Fig. 535 Repair of retinal detachment with silicone buckle. Courtesy of Stuart Green, MD, UMDNJ.

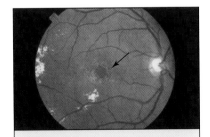
Fig. 536 Diabetic retinopathy with exudates and macular hole (↑).

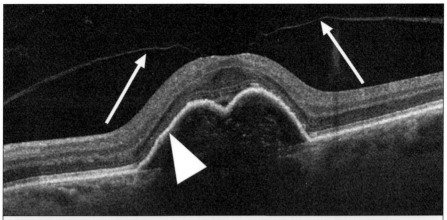

Fig. 537 OCT showing vitreomacular traction (↑) with pigment epithelial detachment (∧) and retinal fluid, but no hole yet. Note loss of foveal pit. Courtesy of David Yarian, MD, UMDNJ.

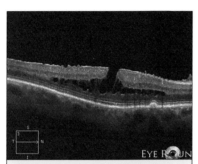

Fig. 538 OCT of partial-thickness macular hole, called a lamellar hole. Also, note epiretinal membrane on surface of retina. Courtesy of University of Iowa, Eyerounds.org.

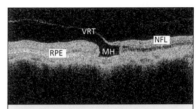

Fig. 539 OCT scan of full-thickness macular hole caused by vitreous traction. RPE, retinal pigment epithelium; NFL, nerve fiber layer; MH, macular hole; VRT, vitreoretinal traction.

tamponades the hole. A newer, non-surgical alternative is to lyse vitreomacular adhesions by injection of a protolytic protein (ocriplasmin-Jetrea) into the vitreous.

Pars plana vitrectomy

Vitreous surgery is performed by inserting three instruments into the eye through the anterior pars plana (Figs 541 and 542). This location avoids the highly vascular ciliary processes, and the delicate retina. The entry

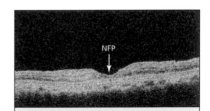

Fig. 540 OCT scan of macular hole resolution after vitrectomy with injection of gas into the vitreous. NFP, normal foveal pit.

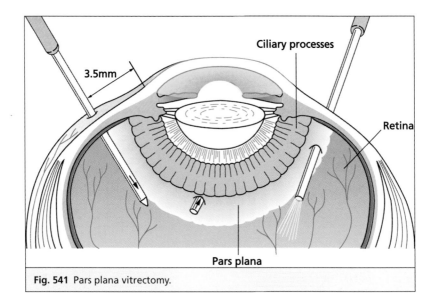

Fig. 541 Pars plana vitrectomy.

sites are located on the sclera by measuring 3.5 mm posterior to the limbus. One instrument is for endoillumination. The second is for irrigation with balanced saline to replace any vitreous removed. The third portal allows for instruments that cut and remove vitreous membranes; obtain tissue for cytology or culture; inject medications, gas, or silicone oil; cauterize or laser photocoagulate the retina; and forceps and/or magnets to remove foreign bodies. These procedures are performed while looking through a microscope with a contact lens on the cornea. Cataracts are a common complication of vitrectomy, followed by retinal hemorrhages, holes, and detachments. Vitrectomy to remove floaters (floaterectomy) is rarely recommended because of these significant complications. For the same reason, a vitrectomy to obtain cytologic specimens is reserved for diagnostically challenging, often vision-threatening, cases of lymphoma, uveitis, and endophthalmitis.

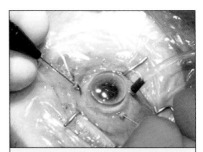

Fig. 542 Pars plana vitrectomy showing sites for illumination, irrigation, and aspiration. The interior of the eye is viewed using a corneal contact lens together with the operating microscope. Courtesy of Stuart Green, MD, UMDNJ.

Appendix 1
Hyperlipidemia

Normal blood lipids	
Normal cholesterol	<199 mg/dL
HDL cholesterol	>39 mg/dL
LDL cholesterol	<99 mg/dL
LDL/HDL ratio	<3.6
Triglycerides	<150 mg/dL

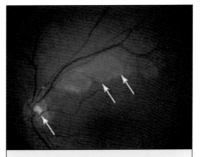

Fig. 543 Branch retinal artery embolus (↑) from cartotid artery and resulting pale ischemic retina (↑↑). Courtesy of Elliot Davidoff, MD.

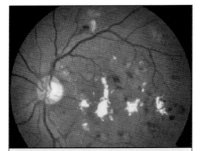

Fig. 544 In diabetes, hard exudates are caused by lipoproteins leaking from retinal capillaries into the extracellular space. Lowering blood fat levels helps minimize this complication. Courtesy of Joanna Gostyla.

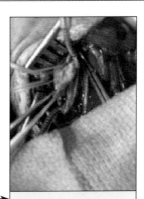

Fig. 546 Thrombectomy using spatula and forceps (see Fig. 135).

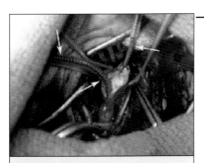

Fig. 545 Carotid endarterectomy showing temporary shunt (↑) to bypass surgical site. It is the gold standard for treating carotid stenosis. If contraindicated, stenting is considered. Courtesy of Niranjan Rao, MD, St. Peter's University Hospital.

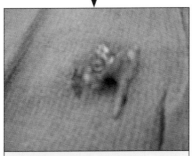

Fig. 547 Plaque removed from carotid artery.

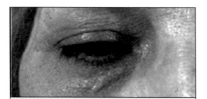

Fig. 548 Xanthelasma are irregular yellowish plaques on the medial side of the upper and lower lids. They are often inherited and sometimes associated with hypercholesterolemia and a 51% increased risk of heart attack.

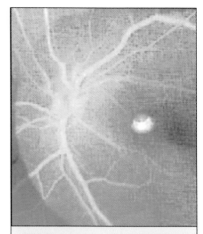

Fig. 549 Creamy, white retinal blood vessels indicating lipemia retinalis which occurs with triglyceride levels >2500 mg/dL. This patient had triglycerides of 29,000 mg/dL and cholesterol of 1470 mg/dL. Courtesy of Murat Ozdemir, MD, and *Ophthalmic Surg. Lasers Imaging*, 2003, Vol. 34, pp. 221–222.

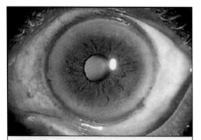

Fig. 550 Corneal arcus is a narrow, white band of lipid infiltration separated from the limbus by a clear zone. It occurs in everyone by age 80. Its occurrence in those younger than 50 warrants measuring blood lipids, which may be elevated.

Appendix 2
Amsler grid

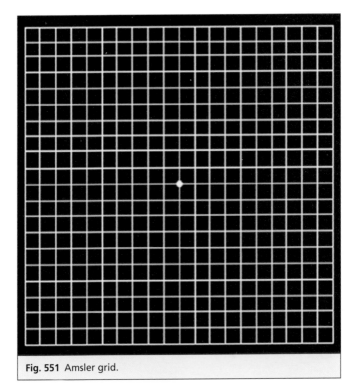

Fig. 551 Amsler grid.

1 Wear best corrected lenses for near vision.
2 Hold card at 35 cm.
3 Cover one eye.
4 Focus on central dot.
5 Detect any wavy, distorted, or blind areas.

Wavy lines and loss of vision often indicate a progression of dry to wet macular degeneration. Lines also become curved in central serous retinopathy.

Index

Page numbers in italics refer to figures.

Manual for Eye Examination and Diagnosis, Ninth edition. Mark Leitman.
172 © 2017 John Wiley & Sons, Inc. Published 2017 by John Wiley & Sons, Inc.

1 If patients complain of blurry vision in their right eye, ask them to cover the right eye. It may be temporal loss on the right side due to a lesion in the left brain posterior to the chiasm. If transient it is most often due to migraine or a ministroke (transient ischemic attack, TIA). Remind them to cover each eye when it occurs.

2 Fibers exit the optic track and go to the superior colliculus to form part of the pupillary light reflex arc, which accounts for the consensual constriction of both pupils when light is shone in either eye.